FROM DOCTOR TO PATIENT

FROM DOCTOR
to PATIENT

Healing Cancer through
Mind, Body and Spirit

DR. DIVA NAGULA

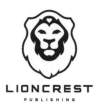

LIONCREST
PUBLISHING

FROM DOCTOR TO PATIENT

Healing Cancer through Mind, Body and Spirit

ISBN   978-1-5445-0374-5   *Hardcover*
          978-1-5445-0373-8   *Paperback*
          978-1-5445-0372-1   *Ebook*

*Front cover photography by Vithaya Phongsavan,
featuring model Gurpreet Singh.*

For all the people who suffer from cancer.

CONTENTS

INTRODUCTION

Rock bottom is further down than you think.

I didn't hit rock bottom when I was diagnosed with stage four non-Hodgkin's lymphoma—at that point I was optimistic, if afraid of the unknown. I didn't hit it when the oncologist told me I needed chemotherapy—at that point, I was furious with God.

I hit rock bottom when I went into remission.

After completing my last round of chemo treatment, I was completely depleted. I was so fatigued that my daily exercise goal was just to walk to the mailbox and back. I had gained weight because I'd been sedentary. It wasn't just my body that was a wreck. During my cancer treatment, I'd become so angry that I'd alienated everyone. I'd exited my business just before my diagnosis, and within the same year I'd divorced and moved to a different city. I'd stopped reaching out to friends, who didn't know what to do with someone who was so sick. I had no willpower, no drive, no reason to get up in the morning.

What was worse in remission was that I didn't have the cancer to be angry at anymore.

My cancer journey had changed my identity. Before cancer, my identity was being a doctor. I had helped thousands of patients in my lifetime. With the news I needed chemo, it was official: I was very sick. My identity switched to that of a patient. Other physicians and oncologists cared for me, but I looked everywhere for answers about how I could recover my health. I didn't feel I could lean on anyone for support; one by one I'd crossed everyone off my list. I isolated myself. It wasn't just my physical body that had cancer. It was also my relationships, my mind, and my spirit.

After the diagnosis, the cancer and I became one and the same.

Then, after five rounds of chemo, I'd beaten cancer. I had been elated for just a moment when the doctor told me I was cancer-free. In the next moment, I wondered, "Who am I going to share this with?" Except for my parents and my immediate family, I was alone.

A few weeks later, I was in a parking lot, out of breath from the walk from the store back to my car. I looked up from the keys in my hand and saw a familiar face coming toward me. *Holy crap*, I realized, *it's Adam.*

Adam was a personal trainer and a good friend of mine. I'd moved to North Carolina for the summer, and after my diagnosis I just lost touch. I never reached out to him when I got sick. He has such a positive disposition, and seeing his face instantly lifted my spirits.

As we exchanged pleasantries, I remembered how great I'd felt when I was working out with him. We would work on strength training and conditioning, but Adam also had boxing pads. Suddenly I said, "You know what? I want to do that again. I want to beat the crap out of those pads."

I wanted to beat up on the cancer and on everything I'd just gone through.

I needed physical exercise, and I needed to release the emotions that had built up over five months of chemo and isolation. I needed to let go of the anger and animosity and mistrust I'd been harboring. I was ready to fight for my well-being.

That chance meeting with Adam started a transformation in my body, mind, and spirit. I was able to reconnect with him, and we had a great bond. My friendship with him allowed me to remove the label of distrust I'd put on all the people in my life. I began to heal my relationships.

As we trained together week after week, my body transformed. Endorphins finally flowed freely to my brain, which improved my mood. I lost weight and my clothes fit nicely. My self-esteem grew as I saw positive changes in my body.

I was filled with hope. Maybe there was a reason I'd run into Adam in the grocery store parking lot. Maybe there was a reason the cancer hadn't killed me. I was given an opportunity to make something of my life. This journey has taught me so much about caring for myself, and I realized my story and my knowledge was now a gift I could offer to others.

In remission, cancer no longer defined me. I began to connect with something bigger than me.

CANCEROUS CHOICES

Chronic inflammation is the root of many diseases and illnesses. In my case, it led to the diagnosis of non-Hodgkin's lymphoma, a blood cancer. For me, chronic inflammation stemmed from poor lifestyle choices such as improper diet, insufficient exercise, high stress levels, and the lack of a support network of friends and family. As I looked back at all the factors that had led to my diagnosis, I realized I'd made myself sick.

As a doctor, I always looked out for the best interest of my patients. But I was also an entrepreneur, stuck in the stresses of growing my business. I had created an unhealthy life-style for myself. I ate poorly. I rarely exercised. I wasn't fully present with my friends and family—in fact, I wasn't always fully present with my patients. I was often somewhere else, trying to get to the next patient, the next procedure, the next development that would advance my business.

I never took time for self-care. I was incredibly hard on myself, constantly pushing myself to succeed and achieve. I never showed myself the love and compassion I needed. My lack of care ultimately destroyed my spirit. I saw the same lifestyle stressors in my patients, and I now have no doubt that these influences had a negative impact on their health— and may be having an impact on yours—as they did mine.

In a typical medical school, doctors are not taught the healing elements of food, positive thought, and spirituality. These are elements I began to learn as a patient and continue to learn throughout remission.

As a student of osteopathic medicine, I was fortunate to learn to look at each patient's disease or problem from a holistic perspective. Most schools of thought focus on symptom management only. From the start of my practice, I took a global view of each patient's physical health. And yet, when I got sick, I realized there was still more to learn.

I looked for alternative ways to tackle my cancer and support myself while taking traditional chemotherapy drugs. I came across a lot of research that wasn't presented to me during medical school. There was much more to learn about health, I realized, than what I had been taught in medical school. While researching my diagnosis and various treatments, I discovered a relatively new field of medicine that seemed to answer a lot of questions for me: integrative medicine. I applied for a fellowship in Dr. Andrew Weil's integrative medicine program, which incorporates elements of Western and Eastern medicine. I was accepted and the program opened my eyes to the healing powers of diet, mindfulness, and spirituality. I also learned that if doctors used the tenets of integrative medicine early on in patients, it was possible to heal people before they developed symptoms and disease.

I realized I could heal myself through my own educational training and personal research.

As I looked for ways to support my health, I also discovered deeper influences that needed healing, from my suffering relationships and Type-A workaholic lifestyle to my mental health and spirituality.

I've been through a number of transformations in my physical, mental, and spiritual health since my cancer diagnosis. For the longest time, I thought I simply needed to eat well and start exercising again. The solution seemed simple. Eventually, I learned that healing also needed to take place in my connection to others and to my spirituality.

I'm still evolving. Through sharing my personal experiences of transformation, I hope to offer a reflection that allows you to develop an awareness of the positive and negative influences in your own life. My cancer is not the only one that began this way. Likely there are disconnections and habits in your own life that are eroding your health.

DOCTOR'S ORDERS

In the wake of a cancer diagnosis, doctors and oncologists give advice on the patient's medical condition—but the patient is left with endless questions about how to support their overall health. Physical symptoms are just the tip of the iceberg, and underneath are all the influences on the patient's well-being: from diet, exercise, and stress to the quality of their connection with themselves and others.

A cancer diagnosis isn't just a personal health crisis. It's a call to develop the unhealthy areas of your life into a more authentic well-being.

In this book, you'll find advice and solutions to increase your physical well-being. You'll learn how factors in your diet, such as eating organic foods and lowering your carbohydrate intake, support your overall health. Supplementation is an important step in helping your body reduce inflammation, and I'll discuss how specific supplements can support a healthy immune system. I'll also share what it's like to get back into physical activity post-chemo, and how important exercise is to your mental health.

As I healed my physical body, it became increasingly important to heal the relationships in my support network. I adopted mindfulness practices and embarked on a spiritual exploration that brought me to an important realization: the health of my mind, body, and spirit affects other people. Negative thoughts are powerful, and they affect others negatively. Positive thoughts and healthy well-being have the power to uplift others.

The purpose of this book—and my life's purpose—is to share the tools I discovered on the journey to better health.

This book is not a replacement for your visits to your primary care doctor, your oncologist, or your psychologist. Instead, it's a prescription for awareness. It's meant to open your eyes and ears to the processes of being healthy, and to use your healthy practices to connect to your deeper spirituality.

Many people who are suffering from cancer feel alone. A cancer diagnosis opens up so many questions—questions doctors may not have answers for—about how to care for and heal oneself. Cancer is isolating because even the most supportive friends and family can't fully relate. This book is a companion and a guide for health before cancer, during treatment, and into a new normal of optimal health for body, mind, and spirit.

Chapter One

SICKLY IDENTITY

Summer evenings when I was in grade school, my dad and I had our ritual: he would get off work, and while my mom was preparing dinner, we would go to the tennis courts and play a match. We started playing when I was eight, and it's no surprise that he always beat me. But by the time I was twelve, I had improved dramatically. I took lessons and played against people with a variety of styles, and competed at a higher level. I wanted to make my dad proud, and I wanted to give him a challenge. Each time we approached the court, I would think, *this could be it. This could be the match where I beat him.*

One particular evening, I could tell my game was different. During the first set I was focused and relaxed, watching the strokes go back and forth, and I slowly realized I was commanding the game. I watched my dad run up and down the court, straining to keep up.

And then, I served an ace. I watched with satisfaction as it sailed through my dad's side of the court, just out of his reach. I'd never done that in a game with my dad before. I looked to see if there was some smile, or shock, or pride—some kind of acknowledgment on my dad's face—but as he tossed the ball back and crossed the court, his face was unreadable.

And then, I served another ace. I won the set.

To put it in perspective, professional players may only achieve six to eight aces in a match. I'd just gotten two, and with the exhilarating feeling of success came a flood of anxiety. I'd won the first set, and I actually *could* win this match. I realized that to beat my dad, everything would need to be perfect.

Instantly, my game suffered. The ease I'd felt in the first set was replaced with self-consciousness as I assessed every move. My mindset had switched—I wasn't trying to win anymore. Instead, I was trying not to lose. I played cautiously. Still, I was keeping up with my dad, and with the last two points to go, it was possible for either of us to win. I really wanted to beat him. I wanted to show him how good I was. Instead, I choked. I double faulted those last two points. My anxiety had gotten the best of me.

I'd never taken a set off my dad before, and so we'd never been tied before. On those summer evenings, we would play two sets—both of which my dad would win—and then we'd arrive home just in time for dinner. This game needed a tiebreaker, but we were out of time.

As we walked to the car, I waited for some kind of acknowledgment from my dad. I thought maybe he'd pat me on the shoulder and say, "Way to go, good job getting that set off me." But we got in the car, my dad turned the ignition, and started driving in silence.

"I can't believe I got that first set," I ventured.

My dad just looked straight ahead. "Yeah, I saw that. You got the first set, but you didn't win."

It was the next challenge, I realized. I wouldn't get his praise until I'd beaten him outright. I realized he would never be impressed simply by my progress; to get recognition from him, I'd have to be exceptional.

Looking back, I can see how this game set the tone for all the achievements I would go on to make as an adult. Later, when my cancer sent my life as I knew it into a tailspin, I returned to these memories to understand how I developed a lifestyle of stress and poor self-care. I'm sharing these stories with you in the hopes that you can see a reflection of your own journey, your own influences, and come to understand a fuller picture of your own health. Mine, as we now know, would end up suffering a lot as I developed and fought off cancer.

The overall state of my health had its roots in my relationship to achievement, and ultimately, my relationship to others.

After that first time I stripped a set off my dad, I kept winning one set but never both. I fell into what became a familiar pattern: I'd choke as soon as it seemed imminent that I would win. I would double fault and give him easy points, and he would win games that I should have won with ease. As this pattern repeated in match after match, I realized that my ego was dictating the game. If I gave my all and failed, that would be far more traumatic to my ego than if I lost through lackluster performance.

My dad's serve was fierce, and it was hard to compete against. I wasn't good at winning the game outright because I couldn't break his serve. But I started to understand that when I put so much pressure on myself to play a perfect game, I always played poorly. I finally decided to take the pressure off. *You're just returning a normal serve,* I told myself. I didn't expect to win, because I'd always lost. Finally, with the pressure off, I played better. The pressure shifted to him to hold his serve, and I watched as he choked. He double faulted at the very end. I won the entire match.

I was exhilarated—I was proud, happy, and mentally exhausted. I'd done the impossible. I was beaming, and I turned to my dad for some kind of acknowledgment and encouragement. But he didn't look at me. I didn't get the recognition I was hoping for. I remember riding home in the car, expecting him to say something. Instead, we drove in uncomfortable silence.

That match signaled a shift in our relationship. I wasn't a kid anymore. I was growing, physically and mentally, into a teenager. This need to prove myself and get acknowledgment from my dad would grow with me, and it would go on to drive all of my achievements as an adult. To fulfill this need for recognition, I put intense pressure on myself to succeed.

It was only later, after my cancer diagnosis, that I'd recognized how much of my life I'd lived in survival mode, and the terrible habits I'd created to support the high levels of stress I dealt with every day. In trying to keep up with my ambition, I would ultimately entrench in a lifestyle that eroded my health a little bit at a time.

THE ROOTS OF AMBITION

Both of my parents grew up in a poor area of India. It's still impoverished now compared to the standards of larger cities in India today. My dad was an only child. His father was not around much when he was young, and his mother passed away when he was born. He left home at sixteen to attend a private boarding school. He was on his own at a young age and he became incredibly driven and competitive at all costs. He focused his life around success, and the path to achievement, as he saw it, was to be brilliant in school. He got good grades and went to medical school. After he finished his degree, he and my mom emigrated to the US because there was a demand for physicians from abroad. He built a medical practice and a surgery center, and he was always pursuing a goal and aspiring to some accomplishment.

The same mentality was instilled in me as I grew up. Even when I was a little kid, everything was serious. Nothing was more important to my dad than studying and performing well in school. That was the mentality of the first-generation Indian immigrants. Especially in the 1970s when discrimination was still present, the only way to succeed in my dad's eyes was to set oneself apart from others. To him, that was the way to live in this country. He felt that being an immigrant set us up for disadvantage, and it fueled his will to succeed and to impart those beliefs to me.

Schooling, culture, and child-rearing are completely different in the US than they are in India. As I grew up, my dad struggled to relate and connect with me, and he didn't understand cross-cultural interpersonal relationships. This presented a huge disadvantage for me. I started getting picked on in school, and I wasn't able to go to my parents for help because they couldn't understand what that was about. There's a five- and ten-year age gap between me and my brothers, so they couldn't help me either. My parents would tell me to ignore it and it would go away, to just study and set the bar higher for myself and I would overcome those issues. They felt if I only concentrated on what's important, I wouldn't have to dwell on those other insignificant issues like bullying and trying to be accepted by peers.

ALIENATION AND ISOLATION

The bullying started in third or fourth grade. Everyone would make fun of me because of how I looked. In India, they styled kids' hair using baby oil. My mom put huge coats of baby oil on my hair, and it was a greasy mess. It was an hour-long bus ride to school, with kids from all grades up through high school. I would fall asleep on the bus with my head against the window. When I lifted my head away from the window, it left a large grease spot from all the oil in my hair. It was a perfect setup to be ridiculed by everyone on the bus, even the bus driver.

The prime target for the bullying against me was my name. My full name is Diwakar, and in Indian culture, the W is pronounced as a V, so my family called me "Divakar." But Americans would pronounce it as a W, so I was called "Diwa-kar" all through high school. Substitute teachers would do roll call, and there was a running joke: when the substitute got to my name, how would they mispronounce it? There would be a long pause after the person's name before me, and everyone would snicker. Most of the time the teacher pronounced it in a way that was vulgar, and the class would erupt in laughter.

I had been happy-go-lucky as a young kid. I would play with other kids, and at home I played with toy trucks and planes, and I'd sing silly songs. But some point, I became very withdrawn. Around fifth grade I started to get down on myself a lot, and I was often disappointed and sad. My parents noticed I didn't hug or kiss them goodnight anymore and asked why the sudden change. I think subconsciously I was angry at them because I blamed them for what was going on at school. Their response, when I would voice a complaint or emotion, was to advise, "Just do well in school. Study, study, study." I started to distance myself from them as well as my classmates. I had pressure from peers at school who picked on me, and pressure from home to do well in school. I was alone, just trying to survive.

Depression settled in. I was enrolled in accelerated and gifted programs at school, but I was not at the top of my class. Social pressures had taken over, and my mind was elsewhere. When I brought my report card home with a D in geometry, my dad crucified me. Worse, I bombed the PSATs, scoring in the twentieth percentile. This would not do: I had to get good grades to get into a good college and begin a successful career path. My dad insisted I enroll in an SAT study program. From then on, studying took over my life.

STUDY, STUDY, STUDY

All I did each day was attend school, do homework, and study.

I memorized the vocabulary section of the SAT guide from A to Z because my verbal score had been so bad. I realized that maybe if I could improve my SAT score, I could have a fighting chance to get out of this life I hated and—maybe—create some sense of happiness in college.

I didn't know what I wanted to do, and my parents were trying to push me into a career path. I considered high-profile occupations: maybe I'd be an astronaut, an engineer, or a doctor. My dad was a doctor, and that seemed like a good lifestyle. The children of my parents' friends were going into medicine, and my dad obviously felt that was the right path to choose.

In eleventh grade, I began thinking about my college prospects. I applied to many medical programs, but there was a specific, new one that my dad wanted me to get into, a college in Richmond. They had an eight-year program that guaranteed acceptance from college into medical school without taking the MCAT, the medical school entrance exam.

The push was on; I *had* to do well. It got to a point where my dad actually studied with me on the SATs after he'd get home from work. This changed the way I focused on school and work. He presented things in a way that was easy for me to understand, and I was able to develop new problem-solving skills in math, and master verbal skills that I'd performed poorly on before. My dad felt if I didn't do well, it would be his fault and we would be looked down upon by people in our community.

For six months to a year we worked on math problems, improving my ability to think and problem solve. By that time, I was sixteen years old, taller, and had beaten him in tennis. He seemed to look at me differently and treated me more as an adolescent than a kid. His approach changed. Instead of yelling and screaming at me, he would work with me, while still applying the same pressure to excel.

With all this preparation, I did well on the SATs—well enough to exceed the threshold needed to apply for the eight-year program. In my senior year, I got a 4.0 for the first time ever. I was on my way.

I was happy about my academic performance, but my social life was still pathetic. I'd never gone out on a date or to parties on the weekends. I was yearning for social acceptance. My focus was just to get myself to college so I could get away from home and start a new life for myself.

I was put to the test and I had to succeed, all for a better future and a better life for myself. It was not about living in the moment in high school; it was all for the future. This future focus kept me constantly achieving and constantly seeking approval. I stopped living in the present.

I didn't take care of my health or the few relationships I had. All my energy went into striving for the next goal. This focus set the stage for my behavior from my childhood on through adulthood, and became part of who I am.

My drive put me on a path that led me to my cancer diagnosis. These behaviors fueled a fire that eventually became my illness.

When I got into that program, it still wasn't enough to impress my dad. It was just the thing that he expected to happen; it wasn't an above-and-beyond achievement. Nonetheless, I think my parents were relieved. I looked forward to college.

I wanted to take the opportunity to see if I could improve my social life. I'd been so focused on being introverted and studying hard that when it came to relationships, I didn't know how to mix with people. I was excited to learn social skills in college. I didn't realize how rough that experience would be.

LEARNING HOW TO HANG OUT

Orientation weekend came, and as my parents helped me get settled into the honors dorm, I just wanted them to go. I wanted separation and independence. When they did leave, I was totally lost. Everyone was talking to each other, hanging out, joking around, and laughing. For the first time, I didn't have anything to worry about, but I didn't know how to be in the present because I'd spent all my time up to that moment thinking about my future.

I didn't know how to hang out with people. I felt the only person I could connect with was my roommate, who was a bit of a weird guy. This guy lacked social skills more than I did. He had a weird, heckling laugh, and spoke in a low, monotone voice. Day and night, he wandered the halls of our dorm in just his underwear. He was eccentric, and people looked down on him for that. I didn't want to hang out with him. There was an in-crowd developing, and I wanted to be part of it.

I decided to change my name and go by Diva for short. I wanted a new identity, to be someone totally different. I intended to leave the old me behind.

At the end of orientation weekend, everyone was hanging out at night, and one of the guys on the floor had a fake ID. He bought a twelve-pack of beer at a gas station and brought it back, and everyone thought he was the coolest guy.

I thought, "Okay, let me drink beer. Maybe that will loosen me up and make me funny." I had two or three beers, and then I became quiet. I was the guy sitting in the dorm room not saying a word. I hated the taste of beer, but every time

I finished one, I'd go to the refrigerator and get another. I wanted to fit in and be cool. Then suddenly it hit me—the room began to spin violently. I went back to my room, four or five rooms down, to lie on my bed. Somewhere along the way, I vomited all over the place. I tried to be as discreet as possible, but some people saw me and made fun of me. After that one night, I was labeled as a lightweight—once again humiliated by my actions and by my peers.

It got better as time passed. I actually became best friends with the guy that bought the beer, and we bonded over watching tennis, of all things. He had played in high school, too. He was outspoken, and girls liked him. He was the older brother figure I never had, and he thought of me as a younger brother. I wanted to be like him. He was smarter and much more confident than I was. He got good grades while I always squeaked by. Our roommates exchanged rooms, and we got to bunk together. We even joined a fraternity together, and I started to meet people. Slowly, I was leaving my social awkwardness behind.

After my junior year, I took an interest in a girl at a frat party. I was about nineteen, and she was five years older than I. I got it into my head that I wanted to make her like me. My ultimate goal was to have her become my first girlfriend. Nothing else mattered at the time. She succumbed and reluctantly became close to me. She was hesitant about the age difference; I couldn't even get into a real bar. For a few months we dated, and my first experience having a girlfriend and feeling those emotions was awesome for me. Life was enjoyable; everything was carefree, and every day was great.

Even though it was short-lived, I was the happiest I'd ever been when I lived in the moment and appreciated everything around me—relationships, friends, life, everything. I didn't realize how important it was to be in the moment. Back then, if I'd asked myself why I was so happy, the answer would have been that I had a girlfriend, but it wasn't really. It was that I lived in the moment. I was in the present, and I was fulfilled.

But then…the school made up a new rule: anyone enrolled in the eight-year program had to have a cumulative 3.5 GPA by the end of the first semester of the junior year in order to matriculate to medical school. I figured out the math: I had to enroll in nineteen credits that semester and achieve As in every one of them to have a cumulative 3.5. My back was up against the wall. I studied and studied. At semester's end, I got all A's and one B. And it wasn't enough.

ACADEMIC DISASTER

With a cumulative GPA of 3.48, I was no longer guaranteed admission to medical school. I had to apply the conventional way. I had to file applications, write essays, and worst of all, take the entrance examination test: the MCAT. I was devastated because I thought I'd had my whole life set. Everything was pulled out from under me; I was reliving high school all over again.

Then my dad found out. Oh my God, I was horrified. He pushed me to get my grades changed. All I needed was one grade changed from a B to an A, in any subject, even if it was a previous semester. We tried everything we could with my teachers. I went to the English teacher who'd given me a B, explained the situation, and asked for an opportunity for extra credit to get my grade to an A. I was not good at English, and she wouldn't change the grade. Then I went to previous teachers who'd given me a B. My dad called every one of my teachers, but we couldn't find anyone to do it.

I had to go the hard way and study for the MCAT. This was harder than the SAT, because it wasn't a matter of memorizing a book. I had to understand core concepts in subjects that were taught from a semester beginning to end.

Then my girlfriend started to hang out in bars I couldn't get into and we grew apart. She broke up with me. It seemed everything was falling apart for me after I'd so recently been on top of the world.

I took the MCAT twice. The first time, I bombed it. The second time, I did better but not well enough. I was approaching my senior year in college, and the future I was supposed to have waiting for me had crumbled. Medical school looked like an impossible avenue for me.

I looked for medical school options that had less stringent requirements. In my research, I came across something called an osteopathic school, that offered a DO degree instead of an MD. They took lesser MCAT scores and the entrance requirements were less stringent. I'd been considering international MD programs that were easier to get into, in the Caribbean or India, but I learned there were schools with DO programs in the US.

I was reluctant as I had never heard of a DO before, but what choice did I have? I applied for a school in Pennsylvania, and my dad traveled with me for the interview and orientation. I was the only twenty-one-year-old applicant whose dad was with him. I was so embarrassed.

As I waited impatiently for months to see if I'd been accepted, I drank heavily to cope. School was no longer important; my GPA didn't matter anymore. I just wanted a break from it all. I felt like things were spiraling downhill and I had absolutely no control over any of it.

For the first time, I felt like my life was out of my hands. My trajectory through school had been predestined; but now, all of a sudden, everything felt like a blank slate. I didn't know how to navigate that, and I desperately wanted to be in control.

When I finally received my acceptance letter, I was relieved: I had my next path in front of me. But I was also burned out and frustrated. I had so many ups and downs, and the only reason for that is that I looked at the end point and not the journey. I was so focused on the goal—getting into medical school and getting approval from my dad—that I went through my early adult life with blinders on. As a student, you know what you have to do to get by, and you don't live in the present day; you live for the future. As I began medical school, that mentality would dictate my lifestyle and determine my mental health.

THE CANCEROUS EFFECTS OF MEDICAL SCHOOL

Erie, Pennsylvania is colder than cold. In Erie, Pennsylvania, there are three hundred and thirty days of darkness and thirty-five of sunlight. It's horrible not to see the sun. As I began medical school, I found myself cooped up in my apartment and back in my old patterns of isolation. I would go from home to the car, from my car into school, then school into my car, and from the car back into the house. I wasn't getting fresh air or much sunlight. It was difficult to build new coping skills. Living alone, I didn't have support from others; but when I was around my fellow medical school students, I still couldn't get support from them because they were going through the same things I was. You would think that in a group setting, you could bond better, but everyone was so stressed out, we were all isolated in our own way.

The schedule was grueling: I was in school from eight to five, and then I would go home and study from six o'clock to whenever I passed out. At the end of the week, I'd go to the bars with my fellow students and we'd all get trashed.

I didn't really have a crowd to unwind with in a healthier way, and it was stressful. I was in study groups, but those social circles were intensely competitive.

At one point, the stress mounted so high that I got in a fight with another guy in my study group. We were going over a topic in biochemistry, and we were exchanging snide remarks as we went over the concepts. No one else saw the meaning in these comments, and they thought it was just good fun. But the jabs cut deep for this guy and me, and we both took it personally. As we kept studying, he alluded to a reference in the past chapter that would have made solving the current problem easier. I said, "What are you talking about?" He responded, "Of course, you didn't know because you couldn't understand the concept."

I snapped. His comment sounded condescending, and I thought he was implying he was better than me. I took extreme offense. I hadn't learned to express my emotions well; when my father said something cutting, I simply wouldn't respond. In school, with the compounded stress, I lacked coping skills. I lashed out at the guy in the study group and initiated an altercation. Neither of us was hurt, but it was the first time I'd started a fight. I was shocked that it got to that point.

Throughout this time, I wasn't caring for my physical needs in terms of getting enough rest and exercise. It wasn't a healthy lifestyle, and it was particularly stressful during exams. We pulled all-nighters, and to keep ourselves awake we drank coffee at 1 a.m. and took ephedrine—a legal substance at that time, but basically a precursor to amphetamines.

I didn't eat well and never had balanced meals. I just ate fast food. The physical abuse of this lifestyle took a toll on my body. I gained a lot of weight, and my body mass index shot into the obese range. Many of my fellow med students went through the same stuff, but the difference was, a lot of them had significant others prior to entering med school, or they found somebody in med school. They had relationships or circles of friends to hang out with. My friends from college couldn't relate to what I was going through. They didn't understand that studying consumed my entire life.

But the unhealthy behavior of my habits never crossed my mind because it was just survival mode. There were no coping strategies taught alongside our rigorous medical curriculum, and it created a perfect storm for disease. I later learned how important a healthy diet, meditation, and rest were for my long-term health. But I knew nothing of these coping skills at the time, and I sorely needed healthy ways to relax.

DESTRUCTIVE COPING STRATEGIES

I used legal drugs to help me study, but they didn't ease my anxiety. I would blow a thousand brain cells binge drinking on the weekends, but I didn't really unwind. And somewhere in the middle of med school, I turned to gambling to relieve the stress. One of my roommates was good friends with a bookie based out of Pittsburgh, and though I wasn't an avid follower of professional or college football, I found it exhilarating to place a bet.

Between school and studying, there was no time to work in medical school, so I was living off of student loans. As I got into sports gambling, it took a toll on my bank account. The bets started off at ten dollars, but as I lost, I would double up to win it back. The bets spiraled to one, two, or even three thousand dollars a bet. It started with football, but as I racked up losses, I started betting in other sports to pay off my gambling debts. I applied for credit cards and maxed them out. My grades suffered because I was worried about trying to pay off the gambling debts. My roommate had been fronting the losses for me to his friend, and he was tired of taking the heat for me. All I could do was apologize; I was broke and stressed.

The debt climbed into tens of thousands of dollars, and I couldn't deal with the monthly bills. I had to call my dad to bail me out. He flew out to Erie and I met him at my uncle's house. Particularly given our relationship, it was one of the most embarrassing moments I've ever had to face. My dad and my uncle set up checkpoints for me to make sure I wasn't wrestling with gambling addiction. I had to send my bank statements to my dad, and he always knew where the money was. He blamed everything on my poor choice of friends, and my roommate who was the facilitator for the gambling. He felt I should be studying instead of trying to build friendships.

The fortunate thing was that this happened near the end of my second year of med school when I was starting to study for part one of my board examination. It was a gut check for me. I normally just did what I had to do to pass because that's all that mattered in med school. You just had to pass, and that's what I did. But the bare minimum required to pass a class might not be enough to pass the boards. To get by, I'd cram the night before a test, regurgitate what I'd memorized, pass the test, and that was it. To pass the boards, I'd have to relearn much of what I'd forgotten. I had to make up for lost ground. Mainly, I didn't want to be embarrassed by failure. That would be a hook, line, and sinker into what my dad thought of me.

I also had to figure out when I could make time to study. Attendance became mandatory, but I befriended one of the roll takers. Somehow this person liked me, and she would mark me as present when she was taking roll. I never went to class, but I used that time to study. Just as when I had the goal of passing the SATs, I focused only on studying. I didn't care about anything else—not my health or my relationships. There was no time to gamble. I was in the zone for three or four months. Fortunately, I passed the boards on the first try.

TRANSIENT LIFESTYLE IN CLINICAL ROTATIONS

The goalposts kept moving: I passed the boards, but the stress still didn't end. The next challenge was to get through clinical rotations. The medical school in Erie didn't have an immediate affiliation with a university hospital, so to fill the clinical rotation requirement, they developed affiliations across the US. We could choose locations based on our proximity or availability, or we could just be assigned.

Everywhere we went, we were alone. The rotation lasted one month or two, and then we switched to another location and started over. Depending on what the institution was like, we'd either stay in a hospital bed or a room that was sectioned off from the hospital. That was our living quarters for a month or 60 days.

I stayed in one place in upstate New York that had subsidized housing owned by the hospital. I had driven eight hours from the previous rotation to get there and was exhausted, but I had to start a brand-new rotation the next day. All I wanted to do was sleep.

I put my bag down, and it was so quiet. It was a two-story unit with three bedrooms and a kitchen, but it was filthy and rundown and no one else was there. I heard something in the ductwork and wondered what it was. When I banged on the ducts, out came a fleet of rats near me. It disgusted me and I ran out of there but didn't know where to go. You had to show up at your clinical rotations because it was part of your curriculum.

I remembered that a friend of mine was from that area and was assigned to a hospital about fifteen minutes away. When I called and told him my situation, he said that he'd be staying with his parents but that he had access to the housing where he was supposed to be, so he met me at 11:30 that night and gave me the keys to his place. I moved in there; it wasn't spectacular, but it was livable. That friend was a savior for me. I got to bed at two or three in the morning and had to show up at six for my new clinical rotation. Every month started like that, not knowing where you'd be living, who your supervising resident was, or who your supervising attending physician was.

Looking back, I'm not sure how I survived it. It seemed the

system of clinical rotation was built without any consideration for our health and well-being. We were being trained, as doctors, to care for our patients—and we were simultaneously taught not to care for ourselves.

THE CONSEQUENCES OF CHRONIC STRESS

The bane of my issues was that I had never been given coping strategies. I lived in constant fight-or-flight mode. I would later learn that sustaining high levels of stress like this can create physiological damage, but it manifests over a period of time. In your midtwenties you may not feel the ill effects of stress immediately. But the cumulative amount over time can cause illness and disease. Additionally, medical students have a high rate of suicide due to the high levels of stress.

I harbored all the stress and internalized it. Visiting my family on occasional weekends was not relaxing. My friends and I had become more distant, a common plight among medical students. I lost what little ability I'd gained to relate to others, especially others outside of medicine. Hobbies and outlets are as important as coping strategies. They shouldn't be something that's discovered at a later stage in life when it's too late.

I began to realize that my fight-or-flight state was so entrenched that if there was a moment of calm, it felt so foreign that I would find some way to stress myself out to feel normal again. I didn't know how to relax or to quiet my mind. If I wasn't stressed out, I didn't know how to function and live.

Getting help for stress requires a support system. In my case, I lacked a network of relationships that could give me sufficient support. I didn't have anyone who could give me an outside perspective and help me understand what was going on. My parents didn't care about anything but school work. I couldn't talk to them about other problems. I wasn't close to my brothers. I had no outlets, and I instead continued to put incredible pressure on myself. That was my survival technique.

In our internship year, we not only had to study for the boards, but we also had to take call. In spite of the stress that plagued all of us, we were on call in the hospital every fourth night. For example, I would work a shift on Monday from 6 a.m. to 5 p.m., then everyone would sign out their patients to me. I would then be on call from 5 p.m. until the following day at 5 p.m. During my on-call shifts, I covered everything that came into the hospital. I had supervision at times, but I did all the grunt work. I'd maybe get one or two hours of sleep depending on how busy the emergency room was. After finally ending what was basically a thirty-six-hour shift, I would crash when I got home. The inconsistent sleep put an intense physical demand on my body.

For the entire internship year, I put in 105, 110 hours a week.

My salary for my first-year internship paid $35,000, which is a great amount of money for a lot of people, but when you consider the hourly rate, it's ridiculous, not to mention the medical school student debt I'd taken on. And there was no way of paying the debts off. My fellow med students and I would just defer our loans until we were able to pay them. Meanwhile, the interest rates were accumulating and compounding.

In an odd way, I think living in the moment during this year kept me from constantly ruminating and having negative thoughts about myself.

I came to recognize the value of mindfulness later, through counseling and training. For years, I had no idea how stressed out I had been; I thought everyone was supposed to live that way. It was a huge revelation to become aware of the stressors in my life and to begin a mindfulness practice to experience life in the moment.

I wasn't happy. I spent those miserable years of medical school striving to graduate so my life could be different. I didn't realize that with my lifestyle choices—eating fast food, sleeping only sporadically, sidelining relationships and hobbies, and putting grueling hours into my career—I was setting the bar for my lifestyle. The culture of ambition had swallowed me, and it was about to get even worse as an entrepreneur.

Chapter Two

CANCER ACCELERATOR

The letter from my first-ever boss was simple and definitive: "This is your sixty-day notice of termination."

I'd just put a huge down payment on a house, and I was being fired from my first job out of medical school. All because of gossip.

I spent an extra year in training to specialize in the new field of pain management. In training, I became friends with a guy thirty years my senior who happened to be a neurosurgeon coming back into medicine after taking some time off. He had some friends who previously worked for him and who wanted to form a symbiotic relationship between pain management and neurosurgery. He proposed that we pair up to make this happen.

It was my first real job with a six-figure salary. I could finally start paying down my debt. I looked forward to my new life, in a new place with new people.

But as soon as I started working for this guy, he began to dictate everything I did as a physician. He scrutinized my every move. Even the way he talked to me was reminiscent of how my dad spoke to me. It was very parental. It got ugly quickly. He and his buddies fed me the difficult patients to deal with, the hard cases that weren't gratifying at all, while he got the great cases. I was the low man on the totem pole. Only five months into this venture, the relationships were tension-filled; it was obvious that I wasn't happy there, they weren't happy with my work, and they didn't like that I was chummy with the employees.

Gossip went around the office about me hooking up with an employee. The gossip escalated until there was too much noise in the office. Naturally, the person who had to be gone was me; I was the expendable person.

My hands quivered holding the pink slip. "Frustrated" didn't begin to describe how I felt; I was completely and utterly stuck.

The clinic was in South Georgia, and the house I'd bought

was a seventy-mile commute away in Jacksonville, Florida. Jacksonville was an up-and-coming city with younger people and a better social life than the small community where I worked, but there was just one problem: I only had a medical license to practice in Georgia. A Florida license was one of the most difficult to obtain, and the process took nearly a year. I had sixty days to figure out a solution.

Someone brought to my attention that a practitioner, who had an office in a small community on the border between Georgia and Florida, was leaving. My boss knew about that, and he'd planted a satellite office in that same region when he gave me the pink slip. I knew his plans, but I figured he couldn't be in two places at once.

I had learned my lesson. I had gone through six months of crap when I was someone else's employee. I decided I wasn't going to be an employee and be told what to do, how to do it, or when. I was going to be my own boss. My medical skills were great. My patients were great, and they loved me. I was performing well as a doctor, but that hadn't mattered. It was the extraneous gossip and stuff I couldn't control that got me fired. I decided that would never happen to me again.

Instead, I was going to be an entrepreneur.

The office management in the new community was lost as to what they would do with their current patients when the practitioner left. They had an immediate need for a physician to replace him. We devised a business relationship that was a happy medium where I could be my own boss and still see their patients and fulfill their needs. Within sixty days, I made this happen and I was so proud of myself. I had no business experience whatsoever, and somehow I put together a business plan, marketing materials, and all the medical equipment needed to start a practice.

My biggest obstacle to achieving all of this was that I needed a loan to buy the medical equipment to perform advanced medical procedures. During my specialized year of training in pain management, I learned advanced spinal procedures that could help patients avoid invasive surgeries. I performed minimally invasive procedures—epidural injections and other techniques—that alleviated patients' symptoms without taking them out of commission for extended periods of time. I had a vision to take this technology to this small South Georgia town and change the whole community.

All of the banks I approached denied me a loan. I didn't have business experience, and I was a risk for them. I needed a $150,000 loan for the equipment and other startup expenses. In order to justify that, I had to show pay stubs for over a two-year period, and I only had a six-month work history.

What was I going to do? My last resort—call Dad. But this time was a little different because he empathized with my predicament. He had encouraged me to start my own business, and he trusted me enough to give me a small loan with the understanding that it wasn't a freebie and I would pay it back down the road when I was able. He loaned me $30,000 in two separate installments, which was enough for me to make down payments and satisfy the vendors.

For the first time, I felt real success. Everything worked out. My interaction with patients was great; everyone was curious about the new technology I'd brought to town. Many were skeptical, but when they tried what I had to offer, they were getting relief. The results of what I did for them spoke for themselves, which had huge marketing benefits. They told their family and friends. In a short time, my business was booming.

BITTERSWEET SATISFACTION

It was an exciting time but also an extremely lonely period because I was by myself. I didn't have colleagues to bounce ideas off of, and I didn't know how to run a business. I never learned that in school. I had to learn about marketing, insurance billing, bookkeeping, and employee management. I had to be responsible for my accounts receivable and accounts payable. On top of this, I still had to provide top medical care to my patients.

I took satisfaction in the fact that I was beating out my competition. My former boss, who had a satellite office down the street, was not doing well there. As I continued to change people's lives and improve their well-being, his demand dropped. He never really got off the ground running because there was so much buzz about what I had brought to the community.

I remember being so happy when I heard he was closing up shop. It was the best feeling ever. I recognize now that there was hidden meaning in this victory: my old boss reminded me of my dad. They were the same age and had similar traits. In all the years of playing tennis, of killing myself studying, of following the path I thought might make my dad proud of me, I never got the acknowledgment I was seeking. I had built up so much anger around how hard I worked to chase his approval and how far away it always seemed. With the closing of my former boss' business, I had a direct comparison: I had succeeded where my former boss had failed.

Even better, I was quickly able to pay my dad back in full for the loan. In six months, I was able to pay my loan off in full. I was so excited to see his reaction when I handed him the check. I thought he would tell me I'd done a good job. I thought he would remark on the success and growth of my business.

But he gave no expression of pride. Instead, he said that in the back of his mind he wasn't expecting that money back, ever. I took this to be very insulting. It was like a slap in the face. To me, this meant that I wasn't expected to succeed and more importantly, not pay off the loan. Suddenly I was an adolescent on the tennis court again, angry that he refused to recognize my achievement.

He advised me to consider moving out on my own, away from the shared office space I was currently in. He was raising the bar to see if I would tackle it. I wanted to define success for myself, but perhaps more than that, I still wanted my dad's guidance—and I still wanted him to be proud of me. I followed his advice. When my contract with that office was up, I opened my own commercial space and hired my own employees. While it was stressful to set up the entire business on my own, within a year everything was on cruise control.

The next year, I pulled my first million. It still wasn't enough to satisfy me.

My business was running smoothly, and I no longer had to stay in survival mode. My mind became idle, and I felt restless. There had to be more to my life than work. I wanted to form meaningful relationships, but I was beginning to realize I didn't have the tools to fix that problem. I didn't know how to form bonds with people.

Instead of working on my relationships, though, I took a

look at what else I could achieve in my business. I could have stayed in cruise control and just counted the money coming in, but no. There was always another bar to be raised. My dad's next challenge: he thought I should build my own surgery center. It's what he had done, and so it was what I should do. I hired a consultant, expanded my building, and began work with a contractor. This new challenge presented so much for me to learn, including the ins and outs of what was required to run a federal- and state-accredited facility. All the money I'd made was going into this new project.

WEALTHY IN MONEY, POOR IN CONNECTION

Building the surgery center was an immense task that took all of my money, time, and more expertise than I had. As we built the new facility, I received a crash course in construction and state certification forms. Perhaps the driver behind it all was still my father: he had set up his own surgery center, and it was the challenge he'd suggested I take on, too. Or perhaps I became absorbed in work and the stress of unfamiliar challenges because I didn't want to face an uncomfortable truth in my life: I was completely alone.

My friendships at the time—if I could really call them friends—were strained relationships with backstabbers and bullies, repeats of the kinds of connections I'd experienced growing up as a child in grade school or as an adolescent in high school. Lacking the mutual respect that comes with true friendship, I built respect with peers in other ways. I achieved.

Money is a status marker, and I watched how people became instantly jealous when I described the year I made my first million. I didn't always wear that status on my sleeve or divulge it in casual conversation, but just having it in the back of my own mind gave me confidence. Money was my way of standing out and gaining respect.

In this way, money was a crutch for my self-esteem, and it was also a boon for me. I took comfort and solace in my achievements; they helped me acknowledge that I was good, and I was OK. Money was rolling in from the surgery center, more money than I had ever dreamed of, and I was investing it smartly. I created a comfortable little bubble, and money gave me greater status that allowed me to feel above people. I hid inside my success.

I could have coasted along on that success, but it would have eventually required me to confront my loneliness. I needed another challenge to raise the bar. My father suggested I expand my brand presence and open a practice in another state, and it wasn't long before I found a potential opportunity in a lucrative practice in Florida. The physician who ran it had fallen ill to cancer and died, and the practice was up for sale by the estate.

At the time, an interim physician was running the practice.

He had also put in a bid to buy the practice. He had built up a huge volume of patients, but as soon as he learned he wasn't going to get the practice, he left and opened up his own business. I had a new practice in another state, and I also had fierce direct competition.

Soon after buying the practice in Florida, I was inundated. The Florida practice I'd bought was already fully up and running, with a full load of patients—all of whom I had to get to know. Simultaneously, I was managing the practice in Georgia, and I was under more stress than ever. Searching for advice, I called my dad.

I expected him to offer suggestions, to tell me what I should do next, but instead he said something I didn't expect: "Maybe you're taking on a little too much."

This idea was so foreign to me, I didn't understand what he meant. I realized later that he was out of his depth, too. I'd already done what he'd done; I'd built my first practice, I'd constructed a surgery center, and now I'd surpassed him by buying another practice in another state. He didn't know what else I should achieve or what other steps I should take.

I ignored his comment, and I hired a physician and a physician assistant to help with the Florida practice. I assumed, like so many entrepreneurs do, that hiring more people would solve the problem. I quickly learned, however, that managing more people creates new problems, and ultimately, it drove me even further away from social connection.

When you hire people to help in your business, you bring on the added stress of managing their personalities. I now had to manage my patients, and I was unable to fully trust my new staff. It didn't take long before I found myself thinking, *screw work, screw people. I hate people.* The thought of taking time to cultivate friendships outside of work repulsed me. I became incredibly introverted.

DIVERSIFYING THE PORTFOLIO OF PERSONAL LIFE

Through my entire adult life, I'd cultivated a single-pointed focus on my work. Looking back years later on these experiences, I realized that there were no outlets in my life. I hadn't diversified my portfolio; I had no hobbies, interests, activities, or people to share my life with. I had no idea the impact this would ultimately have on my health and well-being.

When you invest all your money into a single stock, you're at the mercy of the ups and downs of a lone investment. So it was with my whole life: I lived and suffered by the ups and downs of my business.

It's not just me. Entrepreneurs fall into this pattern all the time. We are devoted to our occupations and we're passionate about our work. Everyone needs passion; without it, there's no drive or motivation. But moderation is required, too. Passion without limitations becomes a full-on binge.

In similar fashion, when I was suffering from work, I binged on alcohol and food. When I went out, I couldn't have just one or two drinks—I'd have five, six, or seven. My whole life was a binge. This lack of moderation meant that when I had stresses in my business, I had no other healthy parts of my life to turn to for support.

When you lift weights, you don't focus on only one side of the body, because the other side of the body will become deficient due to neglect. When you work out at the gym, you want to exercise the left and right sides of the body, so they grow equally and no part of your body overpowers the other. You want balance. I now realize that's how a life should be lived—with good balance.

It was time to work on other areas of my life outside of my business.

THE NEXT CHALLENGE: A NEW RELATIONSHIP

I made one more hire to help create a buffer between me and all the people in my business. I brought in an office manager. In fact, I hired the office manager from my former boss' practice.

I trusted her because I knew her work ethic, and I desperately needed someone I could trust. With her help to manage the people and personalities in my practice, I could manage the structures of two practices and the stress of competition rising around me. It was a constant fight for my volume and my turf.

This woman was nice to me, and our friendship began to develop into a relationship. I gravitated toward her for my sense of well-being and security. My parents had pressured me, since age twenty-five, to get married and give them grandkids. Now in my late thirties, the pressure was even greater. My relationship with this woman was escalating. I suggested we move in together. And then I proposed. She accepted.

Reluctantly, she left her network of family and friends in South Georgia to come live with me in Jacksonville. But she didn't have any friends in our area except for me. We worked together, and then we'd be together at home where the only thing we had to talk about was work.

To add to this stressful relationship, we had a wedding to plan. We were arranging a huge wedding that combined Indian and American traditions. It was going to be in the mountains in Asheville, North Carolina.

My fiancé started to get cold feet. She became distant about planning the wedding and wouldn't help—I thought she was tired, but in reality, she was unhappy. The pressure mounted, and it became too much for her.

A week before the wedding, she called it off.

I was incredibly embarrassed—I'd invited over two hundred people and made down payments on all the preparations—but she had too much anxiety to go through with it.

Up to that point I'd been plagued by work stress; now I was experiencing intense emotional stress. I'd never had a calm lull in my life. This was how I lived—in a constant state of stress.

THE BREAKING POINT

Six months later, she'd moved out, but we were still working together. We got along fine at work, and we were able to keep things professional. To escape my emotions, I would go out and drink.

One day I reached out to her on a personal level and said, "Let's just talk, not about work stuff. We get along fine at work. We play that game. We don't cross each other's paths and that's fine. Let's just talk." We had a really good conversation, and we actually started to date again. She started to initiate things. She wanted to start re-planning the wedding and make amends for the actions she took in calling it off.

As our relationship healed, I finally realized I was done with the stress. My career wasn't making me happy; I told myself that I really hated what I did. I wanted out. I looked for someone to buy me out of the practice.

My old mentor from Atlanta had started buying up practices similar to mine. Most of his buyouts needed rehab, but mine was a successful, well-oiled machine. He made an offer, but a low-ball offer. "You've got to be kidding me," I said. "You should buy me out with enough to where I never have to work another day in my life."

He explained that most times when someone buys a practice, the seller stays on for a few years to ease the transition. I got his point—I wanted out. I took the low-ball offer. I wanted to spend time with my soon-to-be wife because I felt like we were in a good place and things were finally moving in a positive direction.

I was looking to de-stress and turn a new chapter in my life. After six months of negotiating and uncertainty, I finally exited the practice.

It felt *great*.

THE DISCOVERY

On Thanksgiving 2013, I went with my wife to visit my

parents. It was a family gathering with all my brothers and their families. The past few months had been amazing: I'd gotten married, and we'd bought a house in the mountains in Asheville where we stayed during the summers. We took a long honeymoon and spent all of September in Italy. We'd just moved back to Jacksonville for the fall. I hadn't filled my time with entrepreneurial endeavors; instead, I was excited about taking a year or two off, figuring out what I wanted to do, and possibly starting a family.

On this Thanksgiving, I decided to ask my dad about something I'd been noticing for a while in my neck. When I looked in the mirror, I realized my lymph nodes were so swollen I could see them in my reflection. Typically, lymph nodes are small enough that you have to press deeply the sides of your neck to feel them. It was strange.

"Are you sick?" he asked. "Are you getting over a cold or the flu?" We both knew that lymph nodes swell when your body is fighting off infection. But I felt fine. I told him I hadn't been sick in a while. I thought maybe the lumps on my neck were cysts. He didn't know what it was, but he suggested I see a doctor. He sounded concerned.

On my first office visit, the doctor thought it might be a viral infection and asked me to come back in a month, in mid-December. We attributed it to the stress of the sale of my practice.

I chose not to go for that follow-up visit because I wanted to take a couple weeks off and just enjoy the fact that I was not working. It was a great relief; I loved it. When I did go in for a follow-up, the doctor decided I needed to get a CT scan of my head and neck.

He also said he wanted to refer me to an oncologist. I was shocked. *Why the hell would I need an oncologist?* I wondered. He reassured me it was "just in case."

When the CT scan came back, I realized he was right. I did need an oncologist to investigate further. My lymph nodes were all enlarged.

Chapter Three

—∿—

FROM PHYSICIAN TO PATIENT IN A SINGLE DAY

"You have stage four non-Hodgkins lymphoma."

When the doctor delivered this line, my wife was next to me, bawling. I was in disbelief. *I feel fine,* I thought. *There must be a mistake.*

The doctor described what he saw in the battery of scans and tests we'd run. The most definitive evidence for the diagnosis was the pathology from the biopsy of my lymph node. My bloodwork showed abnormalities as well and indicated I had been fighting anemia. Anemia can be seen in people who have advanced stages of cancer because their bone marrow is affected and they're not able to produce red blood cells. My white blood cell count was deficient as well and had been low for some time. These cells are important as they help ward off viral and bacterial infections.

The doctor had a flow chart of specific manifestations and stages of cancer, and he traced his finger across to the specific treatment recommendations. The protocol would be specific to me, depending on my stage, he said. I was in stage four, the most advanced stage. He traced his finger to the bottom of his flow chart and pointed at my treatment option: he felt I would benefit from the most aggressive chemotherapy.

Even though I was a physician, this whole field was as foreign to me as it would be to a patient with no knowledge of cancer.

I did know that cancer is not something that brews overnight. Non-Hodgkins lymphoma specifically develops over years, as cells divide and mutate. This particular cancer is not genetic; it is the result of lifestyle choices. A healthy body is capable of cleaning up these mutations and destroying them. But when your body is triggered and overwhelmed—in my case, suffering from poor diet, lack of sleep, and stuck in survival mode and stress for years—it had trouble removing the mutations. These mutations accumulate, and cancer develops.

MEDICAL CRASH COURSE
THE INFLAMMATION CORRELATION

Among the battery of tests done to determine whether a patient has cancer, oncologists look for markers of inflammation in the blood. In my case, my cancer diagnosis was determined primarily by my CT scan results, which showed enlarged lymph nodes, a lymph node biopsy, which confirmed the pathology, and elevated inflammatory markers in my blood, which indicated that my whole system was working in overdrive to heal.

Our bodies are always trying to achieve *homeostasis,* or a state of stability in our systems. Inflammation is a state in which your body is functioning above the level of homeostasis; it's working overtime to get back to that homeostatic condition. On a cellular level, your body is constantly repairing damages caused by mutating cells, toxins, and other insults to the body. In a state of inflammation, your body is working too hard, and it's not able to recuperate and recover. It's in constant repair mode.

When your body can't return to homeostasis—when it's chronically inflamed—inflammatory conditions, autoimmune disorders, or chronic disease can set in. In chronic inflammation, your body has been working in overdrive for so long that it no longer has reserves to repair new damage.

For example, if I eat a large number of donuts every day, my body has a mechanism to lower my blood sugar: my pancreas doles out enough insulin to return my system to homeostasis. After ten years of donut-eating, my pancreas will have been working in overdrive for so long that it can't produce as much insulin as I need anymore, and that's when diabetes sets in. The body is in a state of chronic inflammation.

Chronic inflammation is typically defined as inflammation that lasts for three months or more. Sustained inflammation over time reduces reserves for repair and leads to disease manifestations.

Risk factors associated with chronic inflammation can include: high emotional and physical stress, chronic infections, smoking, poor diet, food allergies, imbalance of hormones, exposure to chemicals and environmental toxins, poor sleep, and compromised gut function.[1] We will dive into some of these in later chapters.

"Overwhelmed" certainly described most of my life leading up to that point. I'd been leading a very stressful life, a fight-or-flight scenario with no outlets. Even though the specific year after exiting my business was a great year, the stress of previous years of inadequate self-care had taken its toll.

---

1   Roma Pahwa and Isharlal Jialal, "Chronic Inflammation," *StatPearls Publishing*, January 2019.

Poor diet, emotional stress, lack of social support, lack of spirituality, and the rigors of work all combined to create the perfect storm.

Still, I felt physically fine. And sitting in the oncologist's office, he didn't relate how these factors of my lifestyle contributed to the disease he was describing. He didn't describe the impact this diagnosis might have on my mental health, and how I might proactively care for my emotional health.

He walked me through the treatment plan and said he was ordering one more test to confirm the diagnosis. I would need a bone marrow biopsy. This painful procedure was necessary because it was important to know if my bone marrow had been compromised by the cancer.

After we returned from the oncologist's office, my wife and I laid on the couch, trying to figure out what to do. I began researching everything: what therapies are recommended, what the chemo and immunotherapy drugs do, and what to expect.

Though oncology was outside of my professional field, I could understand the medical journals. I read about the outcomes of people with stage four, which at the time, was quite poor. A huge percentage have a relapse within five years, even with treatment. There wasn't enough evidence, for the new medications at the time, to give a positive projection in terms of outcome. Some of the sources referenced a "watch and wait" period among the treatment options, which my oncologist hadn't mentioned. The more I read, the more questions I had.

What was so daunting was not the fact I had to go through cancer and treatment. It was that the life expectancy was iffy—five to ten years at most. That's when it became real to me. At the same time, I knew that cancer treatment comes with high expenses, but it also has a high profit margin for hospitals and practitioners. I wanted a second opinion, and maybe even a third.

SEEKING OPINIONS

I called my brother who used to work at Sloan-Kettering in New York, and he was able to get me in to see a lymphoma specialist. I also made an appointment at the Mayo Clinic with the only lymphoma specialist in Jacksonville, where I was living at the time. Unfortunately, the appointments were two weeks out. I spent the time reading more.

All the statistics said that life expectancy was low because most of the population who underwent diagnosis and treatment were older and didn't have the reserves to fight it. There wasn't a specific subset of thirty-five to forty-year-old patients—they were all lumped into one big category of patients. I wanted to know what physicians' clinical experiences were because they saw patients of all ages and had more experience and judgment than some of the literature did.

By the time my specialist appointments rolled around, I was armed with more information, and many more questions. The bone marrow biopsy had come back, and it confirmed I was at stage four. The Sloan-Kettering doctor, however, disagreed with the potent chemo regimen my oncologist recommended. Because I was younger, he felt I could undergo a less toxic treatment and could possibly get away with watching and waiting for a few months to see how it might grow or regress on its own.

I was relieved to learn I didn't have to go through the most aggressive therapy. The most aggressive chemotherapy drugs make patients sick from the first dose and leave the body so susceptible to anything that patients sometimes die from secondary infections, rather than the cancer itself. Chemo is so toxic to a system that's already fighting to stay alive, that a simple flu, virus, or bacterial infection could create multi-organ failure.

The lymphoma specialist at the Mayo Clinic put me further at ease, in part because his bedside manner was top-notch. He had a good scope of knowledge of the disease, and he was very familiar with what was available in the pipeline for treatments.

While I was concerned about the statistics around relapse,

he was positive. He assured me that there are many available options that are less toxic than chemo. There is a whole family of immunotherapy medications that don't compromise your immune system like traditional chemo does. The doctors at both Sloan and Mayo were in agreement: we would try a watch-and-wait approach.

HOLISTIC SOLUTIONS

During this timeframe of watching and waiting, I continued researching and reading everything I could about different ways of treating my cancer. I knew I needed to focus on better health overall if I was going to maximize the ability of my body to fight cancer.

THE EFFECT OF DIET

I first turned a critical lens on my diet. Before my diagnosis, my diet was abominable. Not counting the scrap of lettuce or tomato on countless hamburgers, I hadn't eaten a vegetable since high school. Since age eighteen, when I moved out of my parents' house and away from my mom's balanced home cooking, I had adopted the Standard American Diet dominated by highly processed and pre-packaged foods. When I wanted to eat "healthy," I'd go to Moe's and get a burrito bowl. Many lunch breaks were satiated by a sandwich from Publix.

I was fueling myself with the Standard American Diet, which

was devoid of nutrients and packed with antibiotics, hormones, pesticides, and chemicals from industrial agriculture. If I was going to watch and wait before resorting to chemo, I needed to focus on better health and maximize my body's functions so it could fight the cancer. The very first thing I needed to do was improve my diet.

If I ate the proper foods and got as many nutrients as I could, I would at least give my body the resources and tools it needed to fight off inflammation and illness.

My research pointed me to three dietary changes that have a huge impact on cancer. I had to eliminate pesticides and chemicals, cut out carbohydrates and sugars, and fill my diet with nutrient-rich foods.

MEDICAL CRASH COURSE
THE LINK BETWEEN PESTICIDES AND CANCER

"Pesticides" is a broad term that includes herbicides, insecticides, fungicides, etc. Studies have linked exposure to pesticides with the prevalence of certain cancers.[2]

---

2   Michael C. R. Alavanja, Matthew K. Ross, and Matthew R. Bonner, "Increased Cancer Burden Among Pesticide Applicators and Others Due to Pesticide Exposure," *CA: A Cancer Journal for Clinicians*, January 15, 2013.

Our immune system is designed to neutralize and eliminate harmful invaders, such as bacteria, viruses, fungi, parasites, and even harmful chemicals like pesticides. In some cases, a healthy immune system can clear pesticides from the body. In those cases, pesticide exposure is benign and doesn't cause much harm. However, when there is a constant incitement of the immune system, such as through too much pesticide exposure, it can be overwhelmed and fail to protect the body from harmful pathogens.

In many cases, pesticides can cause structural and functional alterations of the immune system, which in turn can result in disease. Pesticides can cause overactivity of the immune system, leading to autoimmune diseases, where the immune system mistakenly attacks its own body. Pesticides can also compromise and weaken the immune system, making the body susceptible to viral, bacterial, and parasitic infections, and cancers.

When the immune system is altered and working in overdrive, chronic inflammation can result. Chronic inflammation over time can cause cancer, and I learned in my research that it's a primary risk factor for my cancer. I strongly feel the toxins from pesticides directly caused my cancer or indirectly through its contribution to chronic inflammation.

These effects are so prevalent that Monsanto was taken to

court over the cancer-causing effects of Roundup.[3] We're exposed to these chemicals in our environment; I think of all the Roundup-sprayed golf courses I'd walked in Florida, where I had played golf two to three times a month. More importantly, we're inundated with these chemicals in our diet.

We get a lot of exposure to weed-killing chemicals from the staple crops of the Standard American Diet: wheat, corn, and soy.

These were the first foods I cut out of my diet when I was looking to reduce my exposure to agricultural chemicals, and cutting these also helped me reduce my carbohydrate intake to starve cancer cells. We'll dig into this research, as well as diet recommendations, in more depth in Chapter 5.

In my blood tests, the markers for inflammation were elevated. It was unclear whether cancer caused my inflammation markers to be up, or whether the inflammation had triggered the cancer. Either way, it was clear that to optimize my body and help it heal, I needed to reduce inflammation.

Once I understood the degree to which these chemicals were getting into my steady diet of fast food, burritos, and lunch meat sandwiches, a lightbulb went off: *oh my god*, I thought, *this is why I'm sick.*

---

3   Mike James and Jorge L. Ortiz, "Jury Orders Monsanto to Pay $289 Million to Cancer Patient in Roundup Lawsuit," *USA Today*, August 10, 2018.

I eliminated everything that came from a package or a drive-through window. Even my corner grocery was out—it was stocked primarily with processed foods that contained wheat, corn, or soy. I cut out GMOs and switched to all organic foods (more on that in chapter 5).

I also learned the connection between inflammation and the health of the gut microbiome. My processed-food diet hadn't just been introducing chemicals into my body, but it had been weakening my gut health as well.

MEDICAL CRASH COURSE
THE IMPORTANCE OF THE GUT MICROBIOME

A healthy gut microbiome is characterized by a diversity of bacteria. Even five years ago, not much was known about the role of the microbiome, but as the medical community has turned its focus on gut health, we've learned much more about the importance of a healthy gut microbiome, and the factors that cause disruption in the gut's bacteria.

As you'll see in more depth in Chapter 5, processed food, sugars, and artificial sweeteners have a tendency to kill off "good" bacteria, which creates an imbalance in the gut microbiome. This imbalance of bacteria is called *dysbiosis*: the bad bacteria overpower the good bacteria, and the gut can no longer function optimally, which ultimately leads to increased inflammation in the body.

I eliminated everything in my diet that was devoid of nutrients and ate the most nutritious, colorful diet I could, packing my meals with a variety of fruits and vegetables.

Phytonutrients and polyphenols are important compounds in vegetables and fruits that assist in myriad ways to reduce inflammation. [4] A wide-ranging diet is important for getting all the phytonutrients we need. A good rule of thumb is that the more colors of foods we ingest, the better, because each color of food has a specific phytonutrient that is anti-inflammatory.

I knew the more colorful the food, the more available the phytonutrient content was of that vegetable or fruit. I also began taking probiotics to reduce the imbalance of bad bacteria in my gut.

The next important step was to eliminate sugar. Sugar is fuel for cancer cells. By cutting out sugar and adopting a diet with primarily healthy foods, I could deprive the cancer cells of fuel.

---

4   Swapman Upadhyay and Madhulika Dixit, "Role of Polyphenols and Other Phytochemicals on Molecular Signaling," *Oxidative Medicine and Cellular Longevity*, June 9, 2015.

MEDICAL CRASH COURSE
ALTERING CANCER CELLS WITH DIET

Depending on the cancer, manipulating the diet can have an effect on the proliferation of cancer cells. The majority of cancer cells use sugar as a primary fuel source. In theory, decreasing carbohydrate intake should reduce the levels of sugar in the blood, thus starving cancer cells. However, it is also believed that certain cancer cells can also feed off an amino acid, glutamine.[5] Glutamine is found in protein-rich foods such as whey protein supplements, meat, seafood, dairy, eggs, cabbage, and beans. There are pharmaceuticals in the pipeline designed to specifically block the metabolism of glutamine for treatments of cancer.[6] To optimize diet to fight cancer, it is best to significantly reduce carbohydrate intake and eliminate foods that contain high amounts of glutamine.

That was the theory I was putting into practice: I hoped that by using the correct fuel source and promoting the cells to die, I was finding a way to kill cancer, or at least regress it so I wouldn't have to go through chemo.

---

5   David R. Wise and Craig B Thompson, "Glutamine Addiction: A New Therapeutic Target in Cancer," *Trends in Biochemical Sciences*, 2010, 35(8): 427-33.

6   Tra-Ly Nguyen and Raul V. Duran, "Glutamine Metabolism in Cancer Therapy," *Cancer Drug Resistance*, 2018, 1: 126-38.

I'd never learned these connections between diet and health in medical school, and sadly, no physicians could answer my questions about diet because physicians are not educated about nutrition. That's the unfortunate state of our medical educational system: we learn how to prescribe a drug, but we don't know how to treat conditions with nutrition. Modern medicine treats patients by symptom management, but not by prevention. Diet, I learned, could be a crucial tool for disease prevention and treatment (as you'll see in chapter 5).

Learning this caused me to doubt conventional medicine as a physician. I didn't toss out the whole idea of conventional medicine but espoused the idea of integrative medicine, blending traditional medicine with eastern medicine. There are early measures that can be taken, particularly for individuals with inflammatory conditions, to improve their health and even prevent chronic disease.

SUPPORT FROM SUPPLEMENTS

In addition to diet, I learned about the importance of supplements and began to experiment with them. It began with my questions about vitamin D, which is an essential vitamin to boost your immune system and help your body fight off inflammatory conditions. My primary care physician had never tested my vitamin D level before, so I requested that lab test. The results were surprising: I was very deficient, and it was likely having an effect on my immune system. If

I was vitamin D-deficient in Florida, imagine the population that lives in the north where they stay inside six months of the year.

I was curious about what other supplements might be simple solutions to support my health, and Chapter 6 is devoted to what I learned. Many supplements have great anti-inflammatory effects, and I started taking fish oil, magnesium, vitamin D, and every antioxidant possible to help me fight cancer.

UNDERSTANDING THE ROLE OF LIFESTYLE CHOICES IN INFLUENCING EPIGENETICS

I read about how the new field of epigenetics was expanding scientists' understanding of disease. Think about our genes as hardware, and the way our lifestyle choices influence our genes as software. That programming is our *epigenetics*. By exposing our genes to specific nutrients and lifestyle choices, whether from a vegetable or from emotional stress, we change how our genes are expressed. Those changes can influence many factors in our health and can slow down the growth and mutation of cancer cells.

What we ingest and the physical activities we do can promote epigenetics in a positive way. Proper coping of stress, exercise, diet, and the elimination of processed foods each play an important role. Negative lifestyle choices turn off the genes that prevent cancer and positive lifestyle choices turn the genes on. That was such an eye-opener for me.

As I made changes to my diet and lifestyle, I also saw changes in my body. I lost weight due to eating better nutrients and depriving my body of sugar. My insulin levels were lower; I was eating an anti-inflammatory diet and it was transforming my body. All the excess fat was gone, and I was becoming lean. It was reinforcing to me that these changes were positive changes for my system because I felt better. I wasn't manifesting any of the signs of cancer; I didn't feel sick or have reduced energy. We had moved to Asheville for the summer, and I was exercising by playing golf on a course where I could enjoy the mountains. I noticed I was taking daily naps. I was well rested all the time because I napped for an hour a day and then slept a full six to eight hours at night. It was calming and a good way to live. I wished I had done that years ago. I was enjoying the life I had with my wife.

In fact, we were trying to have a baby. We knew that if I did ultimately need to have chemo, this was our window to try for kids before I started treatment. Chemo chemicals can get into the body, and even affect the consistency of sperm. We knew the pregnancy might not take, or that it was possible to have a successful pregnancy while I was on chemo, but the baby could experience negative effects. We didn't know what that outcome might look like, so I banked sperm in case we weren't able to have a child by natural means. We were unsuccessful, but nevertheless, we were positive about the situation.

I also actively eliminated any negative connections in my life. I eliminated the acquaintances in my life who weren't really true friends. Stress and negative emotions stir up the body's inflammatory state, and I didn't want their negativity to have an effect on me and my health. My idea was to suppress anything that could cause inflammation. I set up my lifestyle to be a driver for positive epigenetics.

My new research expanded my view of how to improve and maintain wellness, and I was on the hunt for ways to regain my health by optimizing my lifestyle. Around this time, I applied to a fellowship in integrative medicine with Andrew Weil at the University of Arizona because it aligned with my new beliefs. The program integrated traditional medicine with alternative medicine—two philosophies into one. I didn't know what was going to happen to me with my health, but this was a field I was passionate about and wanted to practice. This was a way I could help people that aligned with my new philosophy.

NO MORE WATCHING AND WAITING

When fall weather came again and we went back to the home in Jacksonville, it was time for me to get another set of scans to assess what the cancer was doing in my body. I was very nervous about that appointment. I was having issues with back discomfort that I thought was musculoskeletal, but it was near my kidney area and was deep inside. I began having pain with urination, and then the pain in my back became excruciating within only a day or two. I suspected a kidney stone as I had diagnosed them in patients many times.

I checked to see if I could get the scan sooner than scheduled and they were able to accommodate me. When I followed up with the doctor a couple days later, he gave me the unfortunate news that my cancer had accelerated. The pain I was experiencing was due to my kidneys being compromised: my lymph nodes in my abdomen had enlarged and were now encroaching on my kidneys and ureter. I was in total disbelief. I felt fine other than the new pain. I'd been having the greatest six months of my life. How could my cancer accelerate?

The cancer had regressed in some areas of my body, but in others, such as my abdomen, it had become aggressive. I was demoralized. I had studied, implemented, and fought and tried so hard, and now it seemed it was too late for me. I was at stage four when I was diagnosed. Late in the game, I had basically tried to stop the whole cancer progression from taking place. The interventions I'd tried had a positive effect, but I'd only created a small ripple. It wasn't enough.

I needed chemotherapy.

Chapter Four

THE COLD COMFORT OF CHEMO

When you're undergoing cancer treatment, cultivating a positive outlook and caring for your mental state is as important as caring for the health of your body.

Unfortunately, during my chemo treatment, I didn't heed my own advice. I completely shut down.

I stopped fighting, and my mental faculties were taken over by the dark side. I was angry at the world and at life. I hated everything. I was no longer interested in researching what could help make me better—all the research and reading I'd done had gone to waste, at least that's what I thought. I had no more motivation to help myself.

In the back of his mind, my oncologist knew that I would undergo chemo. He was willing to give me the opportunity and the benefit of the doubt to try to slow it down on my own, because I was a physician and was determined to see if I could regress the cancer with my lifestyle changes.

He wasn't surprised that it didn't work. He was more surprised that I lasted six months instead of one or two.

In that sense, maybe my dietary and lifestyle changes did prolong the inevitable a little bit. But I didn't take that perspective at the time; I was angry and pessimistic. Looked at from a broader perspective, I thought at the time, the watch and wait period may have made things worse by allowing my cancer to become more aggressive.

In my mind, it was a failure because my changes didn't achieve what I wanted them to, which was to avoid chemo. During the watch and wait period, I didn't have serial scans done on a weekly basis, so we couldn't tell whether the strategies I was implementing were making the cancer regress, or whether they were ineffective. I think my strategies did help me to an extent, but it was all too late.

My perceived failure angered me for a multitude of reasons. I had to go through the unknown of chemo. I had zero control of the results. I had worked so hard researching, studying, and implementing lifestyle changes and strategies that I did have control over, yet it hadn't worked. I became very pessimistic, cynical, and hateful.

CANCER AND MENTAL HEALTH

My emotional experience could have been modified or modulated if someone had referred me to a mental health specialist. The oncologist at Mayo Clinic had a sign at the front desk of the chemo area, which indicates that a clinical psychologist is on staff. But I didn't ask for that service—I was too angry.

I didn't know at the time how badly I needed it. Issues were beginning to develop between my wife and me because of my anger. I was distancing myself from my family and everyone else. If I'd been given an opportunity to see a psychologist, it may have helped my relationship with my wife and others.

During my years of schooling and entrepreneurship, I had always been driven by competition and my fear of failure. The watch and wait period had been a competition with myself, with the ultimate goal to regress my cancer by any possible means—other than going to chemo. I needed to have some sort of internal drive, because that's how my body was built and how my brain was wired. I was able to look at the positive side of the situation: I knew I had a window of time to change my habits and live. I thought the diagnosis was the universe's way of telling me I had a second chance and that ultimately, if I helped myself, I would have those tools to give other people. I would be able to share everything I was learning about wellness and integrative health, and I'd be able to change people's lives like I'd changed my own. I thought this was the plan for me. I focused on my goals every day: I would build a family with my wife and open an integrative medicine practice to help people with preventative care.

Then everything I had planned for myself went up in smoke.

When I walked into that doctor's office to get the results of the scan, I went from a person who had a planned future, to one second later having all my hopes, wishes, and dreams vanish. I was angry with God.

Suddenly I felt alone and hopeless. Everything I had envisioned for myself crumbled. I didn't even know how to live the next day. I couldn't take one day at a time because that was so foreign to me. I wasn't scared of dying; I was pissed that I had failed. There were so many things I could've done and wanted to do, but they hadn't been in my focus before. As a result, my anger escalated.

My question wasn't, "Why me?"

It was, "What now?"

I was done; I had nothing left to fight.

CHEMO BEGINS

Everyone's experience with chemotherapy is a little different depending on what cocktail they're given for their type of cancer. My cocktail was not as potent as some other options, but definitely more potent than others. I received a combination of chemotherapy and immunotherapy to battle my cancer, and my treatment happened once a month for six months. Each treatment involved a two-day session: the first day I received an eight-hour infusion, and the second day I received a four-hour infusion. I sat in a chair the whole time these drugs were being infused into my body.

MEDICAL CRASH COURSE
CHEMOTHERAPY AND IMMUNOTHERAPY

Chemotherapy refers to the medications typically used to blast cancer cells. The disadvantage is that these drugs affect good cells along with the bad.

Immunotherapy is medication that enhances the immune system to fight cancer by targeting specific cells. Some cancers are more susceptible to immunotherapy, while other cancers are only susceptible to chemo. Now, researchers are finding that a combination of immunotherapy and chemotherapy together fights off cancers more than just one modality alone.

There are a growing number of services that cancer patients can use to have their tumor cells tested. **Personalized Cancer Treatments** can produce an individual profile based on tissue samples and genetics and provide information about what drugs and natural substances are most effective in treating the specific cancer.

Many people have a misconception that all chemotherapy leads to hair loss, weight loss, nausea and vomiting, and malaise. My chemo experience progressed in a gradual manner. The immediate exposure to chemo was toxic itself, but it took a while to act on my system.

Additional doses are what made the medicines more toxic to my body.

As I was exposed to chemo medicine over the course of six months, I felt the effects more and more. The first week after my first treatment was when my nausea was the worst; then it subsided. The main effects I experienced were low energy and an inability to focus. I had a constant state of brain fog and lowered mental capacity. In addition, I actually put on weight because I was very sedentary with no energy to exercise. Just to get from my front doorstep to the mailbox and back had me huffing and puffing.

UNINTENDED RIPPLE EFFECTS

During chemo, my mental state was compromised because I just gave up. I shut down emotionally and mentally, and I didn't put up enough of a fight against the cancer. My negative outlook created ripple effects beyond my physical healing; my relationships suffered, and my support network collapsed.

I had shut myself off, and my wife didn't know how to deal with that. We had a major lack of communication. That we were struggling to talk to each other should have been a sign that we needed help from a therapist. A lot of miscommunication and other issues could have been resolved if we had better communicated our feelings. Our relationship suffered so much that we ultimately got divorced.

If I'd had a more positive mindset, it would've allowed me to be more open to having better relationships with others. My parents called me incessantly, two or three times a day, asking how I was doing. They wanted to visit me often, but I didn't want that—I didn't want to be reminded that I was sick. If I'd been more positive, I would have probably looked at it in a different way. I would've recognized that people cared about me and wanted the best for me.

In this period where I was angry at God, anger was all I could see. It was only later, after I adopted the spiritual practices you'll read about later in this book, that my positive outlook and my overall health began to change.

The start of chemo marked the beginning of the darkest part of my life. Looking back, I can see clearly that there were several measures I could have taken to practice better self-care during this period. Research and my own experience have taught me better ways to support my wellness during an intense health crisis, and I hope that if you are undergoing chemotherapy, you'll find the following suggestions helpful for your own self-care.

SUPPORTING HEALTH DURING CHEMO

It's helpful before starting chemo to prepare yourself physically as best you can. Chemo has the potential to reduce your mobility, and the better shape you can be in prior to the state of potential immobilization, the better for your body to handle any illness or insults to which it will be exposed. It's easier to prepare your body while you're in a pre-chemo state.

Exercise, walk, and perform as much physical activity as you can without causing harm to your body. During chemo, walking is the easiest way to maintain physical activity. You don't have to get on a bike and go for miles on end. Any sort of physical activity you can manage where your body is moving is beneficial. You'll circulate blood in your system and stimulate your lymphatic system, which will help facilitate the removal of toxic by-products from chemotherapy. It will also help circulate oxygen and vital nutrients that your body needs. Maintaining physical exercise is sometimes easier said than done, because some people are bedridden and are so physiologically incapacitated by chemo.

Always drink a lot of fluids, which help flush out toxins. Stay hydrated. Eat as much as you can tolerate of healthy and balanced nutrition.

A lot of supplements help fight off cancer, but deciding whether to take them during chemo can be complicated. You want the chemotherapy to work, and taking supplements in conjunction with chemo could interfere with chemo's cancer-fighting effects on the body. You need to be judicious about what you take, and make sure to disclose any supplements you take to your physicians.

CARING FOR YOUR MINDSET

Most importantly, take care of your mental health. There is a mental and emotional aspect to chemo that patients and doctors don't often talk about. In my case, which was not unique, I was left in a state of hopelessness, which is the worst state a person could be in while undergoing treatment for cancer. When the prognosis of your disease is uncertain, you can't plan anything from one day to the next. You don't know what to expect—in terms of how you'll feel each day, or in terms of the course of the disease.

A positive mindset is crucial. You must actively want to get back to where you were before the cancer. Thinking positively has a beneficial effect on your stress levels, and on the cancer itself. With a positive mindset, you will notice and attract positivity around you. A negative mentality attracts negativity. Having a positive mindset and expecting good outcomes has a huge impact on how much success you'll have in beating cancer and returning to a better quality of life.

It's helpful to work with a therapist to support your mental health and outlook while undergoing cancer treatment. Oncologists often have cancer psychologists or oncology social workers as a part of their team, particularly if they're working with an academic institution. Cancer therapy wasn't recommended to me; with my background as a physician, my doctors may have put me in a category where they figured I knew what to do. I didn't.

Unfortunately, when you're dealing with a difficult situation like undergoing cancer treatment, you can't see it from an outside perspective. It's difficult to catch your own negative mental patterns. The cycle just spins in circles, and therapy can help you develop strategies to break it.

A therapist can help people see the effects the cancer journey has on their mental well-being and their relationships. Your relationships with your spouse, close friends, and family members are affected by your mindset. Therapy can help a patient develop better communication skills with the people in their support network and strengthen those relationships. I believe that receiving counseling could have possibly saved my marriage. I definitely would have benefited from a recommendation to an experienced counselor and would advise the same for anyone else going through cancer.

As a patient, be proactive and ask your physician for recommendations for grief counseling. If you're skittish about opening a phone book or doing a Google search, your physician will definitely have recommendations.

Undergoing cancer treatment can take a physical and mental toll on your body, but there are steps you can take to support your body and your mind. What I needed most in my cancer journey was support for my physical, emotional, and spiritual health. Before chemo, I had made some lifestyle changes in an effort to reduce my cancer. While these changes hadn't stopped the course of my cancer, they had created positive changes for my overall well-being. After chemo, I realized I had an opportunity to bring all these areas of my life back to wellness. I returned to all the healthy habits I had begun in the watch-and-wait period and adopted new practices as I learned better ways to optimize my lifestyle—practices you'll see in detail in the next chapters. Chemo had brought me to the lowest point of my health and my life. I hoped I could have a whole new level of health in remission.

Chapter Five

FEED THE SOUL, STARVE THE CANCER

Before I was diagnosed with cancer, you could have summed up my version of the Standard American Diet as "anything that was not green." I knew McDonald's was terrible, but I considered Chik-fil-A to be a healthier option. Of course, we now know how that turned out.

The major hallmark of the Standard American Diet is that it is made up of processed foods that are devoid of nutrients. The whole point of eating food should be to have nutrition that can help you fight disease, reduce inflammation, and provide you with nutrients to promote a healthy lifestyle. A healthy diet includes whole foods: nuts, vegetables, fruit, lean meats, and whole grains.

As I researched the connections between diet and cancer, I also learned that diet impacts the overall health of our gut—which then has an effect on our immune response. My diet, as it turned out, was disrupting my gut microbiome, promoting inflammation throughout my body, and fueling my cancer.

MANAGING OUR MICROBIOME

About a hundred trillion organisms colonize our gut, specifically the portion in the lower part of the colon. These microorganisms are collectively known as the human gut microbiome, and they function as cofactors that assist with our bodily processes. Our "gut" includes our small and large intestines, which are responsible for absorbing nutrients from our food and eliminating waste. They accomplish this with the help of bacteria that break down our food by unbinding substances that we ingest and allowing appropriate vitamins and other nutrients to be released. These bacteria also allow our body to detoxify, by binding harmful chemicals to be eliminated.

With so many important functions, the microbiome can protect us from disease or make us sick. It's important to treat our gut bacteria as best as we can. Simply put, we provide them with food to flourish, and in turn, they serve us in various ways. When we have an optimally functioning gut, we have a wide variety of good and bad bacteria. Through the food we ingest and through our environment, our gut is exposed to bad viruses, bacteria, and fungus. A healthy supply of good bacteria serves as our first line of defense against foreign invaders. Our gut bacteria help regulate immunity and assist in fighting inflammation—which can help protect us against cancer.

An optimal gut microbiome is necessary to help cancer patients recover from chemo or radiation. These treatments kill cancer cells, and they give the gut and the immune system a lot to process and clean up. When we don't have proper gut bacteria, we may not be able to take advantage of the healing effects of these therapies.[7]

Ideally, you want to have the good bacteria outweigh the bad. This mix of bacteria is supported by what we eat: the good bacteria thrive with whole foods, and the bad bacteria thrive with processed, sugar-laden foods. Through our diet, we can create a healthy environment for our good gut bacteria and prevent disease states such as cancer and autoimmune conditions.

The gut microbiome has been a hot research topic in recent years, and researchers are discovering that a lot of our well-being is determined by the integrity of our gut health. The gut is a second brain, and the activity of good bacteria improves

---

7   Muhammad Hassan Raza, et al, "Microbiota in Cancer Development and Treatment," *Journal of Cancer Research and Clinical Oncology,* December 5, 2018.

our immune system and brain functioning. Specific strains of our gut bacteria produce "feel-good" neurotransmitters such as dopamine and serotonin to regulate our mood and behavior. When a person is anxious or depressed, it's often due to an imbalance of neurotransmitters. By focusing on the health of the gut, it's possible to restore these neurotransmitters to balance through natural methods. In promoting our gut health, we create a whole host of benefits for our bodies and minds.[8]

Conversely, when our diet contains too much sugar and not enough nutrients, we skew the balance of bacteria in our gut. When bad bacteria begin to overtake the good, it leads to *dysbiosis* in the gut.

MEDICAL CRASH COURSE
THE DAMAGE OF DYSBIOSIS

The bacteria in our gut are kept in balance by constant competition between the different strains. In a healthy microbiome, the good bacteria dominate. But when the balance is disrupted—by poor diet, environmental toxins, or antibiotics—bad bacteria can begin to win out in the competition. This prevalence of bad bacteria is known as *dysbiosis*.

---

8   Francis Okeke, Bani Chander Roland, and Gerard E. Mullin, "The Role of the Gut Microbiome in the Pathogenesis and Treatment of Obesity," *Global Advances in Health and Medicine*, May 2014, 3(3): 44-57.

If your gut is in a persistent state of dysbiosis, *leaky gut syndrome* can result. Leaky gut occurs when an insult to the delicate gut lining (such as an imbalance of gut bacteria) causes inflammation of the gut tissue, leading to alterations of permeability. That increased permeability results in movement of toxins and gut bacteria into the bloodstream. These "leaks" in the gut lining can lead to altered absorption of essential food nutrients. Foreign molecules can be absorbed into the bloodstream, causing the immune system to create more antibodies to neutralize and eliminate them. Because the immune system is in overdrive, leaky gut can increase susceptibility to viral and bacterial infections and can be the source of chronic allergies and gastrointestinal problems.[9]

Although some diseases may not appear to be related to gut health, all disease states, whether heart disease, allergies, or cancer, are, in essence, an enhanced inflammatory state. There is a spectrum of inflammation, and if we don't have a proper balance of gut bacteria, we are unable to regulate our inflammatory state, and we leave ourselves prone to health issues, be they something fixable or chronic. I believe that it is the disruption of the gut microbiome that contributes to a lot of health issues, including cancer, that we see today.

The balance of the microbiome is disrupted on a regular basis in a variety of ways, from exposure to Roundup and other chemicals in processed foods, to livestock that are injected

9   Catherine Guthrie, "How to Heal a Leaky Gut," *Experience Life*, March 2015.

with hormones and antibiotics, to the antibiotics we're prescribed to deal with an infection. It's possible, however, to repair these effects by adopting healthy diet and lifestyle habits that promote the health of our gut.

HOW TO KNOW IF YOU HAVE DYSBIOSIS

Dysbiosis and leaky gut are conditions that result from the cumulative effect of lifestyle choices. Eating pizza one day a week may not cause issues, but after eating pizza three times a day for twenty years, your microbiome may certainly be affected, and your immune system may have trouble keeping up.

Dysbiosis manifests in bloating, cramping, and gas, and it's important to be in tune with those symptoms. Other systemic issues may signal an imbalance in the gut, such as being more susceptible to bacterial and viral infections. Being sick is a result of an immune system that is not functioning optimally. Taking antibiotics to treat disease also impairs your gut because they unbalance the microbiome, often killing off the good bacteria along with the bacteria causing the infection. If you're getting sick frequently, you can reverse-engineer the cause: could it be in the gut?

You can correct dysbiosis by eliminating processed foods and eating fruits, vegetables, and most importantly, fiber. Fiber feeds the good bacteria, and it's typically absent from processed foods. Taking probiotics is also helpful, but the good bacteria won't prosper without being fed fiber. You can't fix the problem overnight, or with just a pill. Instead, you need to feed your microbiota the foods that allow good bacteria to flourish naturally, and limit the foods that cause bad bacteria to thrive.

A HEALTHY GUT BEGINS WITH DIET

My first step in promoting a balanced microbiome and regaining health was to cut out processed foods and replace them with fresh foods.

Processed food is specifically any food that's been altered in some way during preparation. This can include freezing, canning, baking, and dyeing the food. The resulting processed foods contain higher levels of salt, sugar, and saturated fat that counter their nutritional value. In addition to excessive calories, processed foods contain additives that extend their shelf life. A can of Coke is a prime example of a processed drink with no beneficial nutritional value. It's not natural, is high in calories, and it contains additives. (In addition to all of that, it is highly addictive.)

Fast food, packaged and canned food, processed meats, and refined grains all fit into the category of processed foods. Simply by filling my diet with whole foods, I was eliminating a lot of additives and packing more nutritional value into my meals.

My next task was to eliminate simple carbohydrates. As we discussed in Chapter 3, cancer cells feed off of sugar and glutamine, and by cutting my sugar intake and eliminating glutamine-rich foods, I knew I would be able to help facilitate cell death in cancerous cells.

OPTIMIZING DIET DURING CANCER

As I discussed earlier, we want to do our best to starve cancer cells and if we undergo chemotherapy, we want to optimize its effects, and starving the cancer cells of its fuel helps facilitate the effects of chemotherapy.

The first step to cutting sugar-rich food, the cancer's primary fuel source, is to eliminate all refined sugar products, all refined foods (white flour products, white rice), and fruit juices, which contain high levels of sugar and high fructose corn syrup without the necessary fiber we naturally get from eating whole fruit. That morning donut and afternoon can of Coke are obvious culprits to avoid. Read labels and throw out any products with flour or sugar in their ingredient lists. Consumption of desserts and other rich foods allow the cancerous cells to be exposed to sugar, which feeds their growth.

It's almost impossible to eliminate carbohydrates from your

diet altogether; fresh fruits and vegetables count as carbohydrates, but we don't want to eliminate those; their nutritional value and phytonutrient content are beneficial to our bodies.

We also have to address cutting out cancer's secondary fuel, glutamine. Glutamine is an amino acid and it can be found in many protein-rich foods. It is the most abundant free amino acid in the blood. Consumption and processing of glutamine sustains cell growth and proliferation. Glutamine brings nitrogen to the cancer cells so they can use it to make essential amino acids, and thus the proteins required to make more cancer cells. Cancer cells can become addicted to glutamine, thus targeting the metabolism of glutamine has been recently developed as a strategy against cancer.[10] Eliminate glutamine-rich foods such as red meats, wheat, and all dairy products except cottage cheese.

As I determined which foods to include in my diet, I automatically eliminated all red meats, flour products, all types of sugars, and of course, sweets. When it came to whole foods that contained sugar, such as fruits, I paid attention to how those foods affected my blood sugar levels. To do this, I looked to foods that were low on the *glycemic index* and that had a low *glycemic load*.

---

10   Tra-Ly Nguyen and Raul V. Duran, "Glutamine Metabolism in Cancer Therapy," *Cancer Drug Resistance*, September 19, 2018, 1:126-138.

MEDICAL CRASH COURSE
FOLLOWING THE GLYCEMIC INDEX AND
UNDERSTANDING GLYCEMIC LOAD

One way to assess the impact of carbohydrates is to look at how different foods affect blood sugar levels. How much a food spikes your blood sugar level is measured by its *glycemic index*. A quick internet search will pull up huge lists ranking the glycemic indexes of all kinds of foods—from the sugar high of a bowl of ice cream to the negligible effect of a stick of celery. Eliminate foods that spike blood sugar on the high end of the spectrum and stick to foods with a low glycemic index.

In healthy individuals, consuming low-glycemic foods allows fewer opportunities for the sugar to be stored as excess fat. In cancer patients, you want to eliminate processed sugar and eat fruits and vegetables. By choosing fruits and vegetables with low glycemic indexes, you are minimizing sugar consumption while preserving adequate phytonutrients to reduce inflammation.[11]

Glycemic load gives a more complete picture of a food's impact on blood sugar by accounting for the amount of carbohydrate in a single serving size. It is calculated by

---

11   M. L. Neuhouser, et al, "A Low-Glycemic Load Diet Reduces Serum C-Reactive Protein and Modestly Increases Adiponectin in Overweight and Obese Adults," *The Journal of Nutrition*, 2012, 142(2): 369-374.

the following formula: GL = GI/100 x net carbs where net carbs are equal to the total number of carbohydrates, minus dietary fiber.

By eating a diet of whole grains, fruits, and vegetables, you increase the amount of fiber in your diet and subsequently lower your glycemic load. A 2012 study showed that a low glycemic load diet was associated with a reduction in inflammatory blood markers (C-reactive protein, or CRP) in individuals with elevated body fat.

WHAT TO EAT

The anti-inflammatory diet, keto diet, paleo diet, and Mediterranean are all examples of healthy eating plans. They don't contradict each other, and the basic fundamentals of these diets are to keep the glycemic index low and eliminate processed foods. They focus on vegetables, lean meats, fruit, healthy fats, and in some cases, whole grains. Such diet habits have been shown to promote healthy living and to reduce cardiovascular disease and obesity. I don't espouse a specific diet, but these are all good options for your own further research. When you've established what your dietary goals are, you can pick and choose what to follow from these diet recommendations.

Not every diet works for everyone. Some of the components of these diets are too broad, and need to be tailored to the individual's needs, particularly for people who are dealing with cancer. For example, the paleo diet may not be appropriate for a person suffering from cancer because there are high amounts of glutamine-rich foods in the form of lean meats. If you have been diagnosed with cancer, it is a good idea to speak to a dietitian or physician to see if you would benefit from eliminating sugars and/or glutamine-rich foods.

There is a benefit to each of the diets described next, but the question is whether or not the diet can be sustainable for you. For this reason, diet should be tailored to each individual person according to what works for them.

KETOGENIC DIET

A basic ketogenic diet consists of lean meats, high healthy fats, and low carbohydrates, typically around 50 grams per day or less, that come from vegetables and fruits. With a low intake of carbohydrates, the body stays primarily in ketosis, which breaks down fat for fuel, helps regulate blood sugar levels and fights inflammation. Ketosis in itself produces anti-inflammatory benefits, which is important for a person who is proactive about preventative practices. Being in ketosis has been shown to prolong life.[12]

---

12   Nate Martins and Dr. Brianna Stubbs, "Keto Diet Fundamentals," *HVMN*, February 19, 2019.

PALEO DIET

The focus of the Paleo diet is to eliminate all processed foods. The guidelines are simple: in this diet, you eat as hunter-gatherers did. This means sticking to foods that were grown on the ground or in the ground, or animals that feed off of the ground. Grains are eliminated because while they grow from the ground, they have to be processed to be edible. There is no restriction on the amounts of meat and vegetables you eat, and because of the elimination of grains, this is generally considered a low-carb diet, although the carbohydrate intake is not as restricted as with a ketogenic diet.

ANTI-INFLAMMATORY DIET

Dr. Andrew Weil, the program director for the integrative health fellowship I joined during my cancer journey, came up with the anti-inflammatory diet, which is designed to moderate inflammation.[13] He points out specific foods, such as particular vegetables, fruits, beans, grains, organic lean meats, and mushrooms, that should be eaten regularly for their anti-inflammatory effects. These foods are rich in anti-oxidants, polyphenols, and vitamins, which help the body reduce inflammation.[14]

The key is to keep this diet clean by avoiding processed

---

13   "Dr. Weil's Anti-Inflammatory Diet," Weil, 2019.

14   Swapna Upadhyay and Madhulika Dixit, "Role of Polyphenols and Other Phytochemicals on Molecular Signaling," *Oxidative Medicine and Cellular Longevity*, June 9, 2015.

foods, promoting whole grains and whole foods, and vary the content of your diet on a regular basis to allow exposure to different nutrients, phytonutrients, and polyphenols. This diet does have carbohydrates, but they are low-glycemic carbohydrates such as whole grains. The anti-inflammatory diet espouses 200-300 grams of carbohydrates per day, and that's probably too high for a person in a state of cancer; for someone actively looking to manage a state of cancer, the ketogenic diet may be a better choice.

MEDITERRANEAN DIET

The Mediterranean diet is a combination of all of these and involves eating a lot of healthy fats like olive oils, nuts, almonds, and lean fish. These fats contain high levels of omega 3's, which are anti-inflammatory. In addition, the high level of fat in this diet helps you feel more satiated because you feel full.

CUTTING OUT CHEMICALS

In addition to paying attention to which foods you include in your diet, it's important to look at the quality of your food. We saw the connection between pesticides, weed-killers, and cancer in Chapter 3. These chemicals are prevalent in our conventionally grown foods; the fruits and vegetables in the produce section of your typical corner grocery store have been sprayed repeatedly with herbicides and pesticides to enhance growth efficiency and to ensure that no weeds affect the crops. One of the big culprits is Roundup, which contains the chemical glyphosate. The FDA recently labeled glyphosate carcinogenic, and yet, Roundup is nearly omnipresent in modern-day farming.[15] Farmers want a high yield, so they use pesticides and herbicides heavily.

Over time, these chemicals can accumulate in the body and become toxic. By eating organic, you can reduce your exposure to pesticides and increase the antioxidant content of the food you ingest. Additionally, it makes for better-quality food that also tastes better. Ideally, you want to take your diet a step further and eat all organic and non-GMO foods to reduce the amount of these chemicals you consume.

MEDICAL CRASH COURSE
GMOS EXPLAINED

At least 90 percent of the United States' staple crops, such as corn, soy, cotton, canola, and sugar beets have been genetically engineered. A genetically modified organism (GMO) is the result of this engineering process where genes from the DNA of one species are extracted and forcefully inserted into the genes of an unrelated plant or animal. The foreign genes may come from bacteria, viruses, insects, animals, or humans.

---

15   Dr. Joseph Mercola, "Go Organic," *Mercola*, January 9, 2018.

The purpose of this technology is to be able to transfer a desired trait found in nature from one organism to another. For example, the above-mentioned crops have been genetically modified to be glyphosate-resistant. As a result, there is an increase in glyphosate use, which has led to the development of glyphosate-resistant weeds (superweeds), all negatively impacting the environment and human health. An increase in chemical use on these crops, of course, means an increase of these chemicals in our food. Our exposure to these chemicals is much higher with GMO-ready crops.[16]

Conventionally raised meats also contain these chemicals, which are found on the grains that are fed to livestock. If you eat beef, you should eat meat that is organic and grass-fed. Conventional livestock are given synthetic growth hormones to increase lean muscle mass and produce more milk. These animals are often given antibiotics to control for diseases, since they are often raised in unsanitary conditions, so the animals can be quickly sold and butchered.[17] These hormones and antibiotics disrupt our gut's microbiome. Hormones in conventional meats compromise our endocrine system, and the antibiotics in meats not only disrupt our gut bacteria, they can also cause our bodies to develop antibiotic resistance. Antibiotics kill all of our gut bacteria, good and bad, leading to poor gut health and dysbiosis.

---

16   "GMO Facts," *Non-GMO Project*, 2018.

17   Amanda Macmillan and Julia Naftulin, "4 Science-Backed Health Benefits of Eating Organic," *Time*, July 27, 2017.

The effects of these chemicals are so great that a 2018 study in France found that eating organic foods can reduce your likelihood of acquiring a cancer. The researchers followed a group of 70,000 individuals, dividing them into a group that regularly ate organic foods, and a control group that did not. The organic-food group had an overall reduction in cancer incidence by 25 percent—and a 73 percent decrease in cases of lymphoma.[18]

An earlier 2014 study in England showed a different set of results, namely, that there wasn't any significant correlation with organic food and overall cancer reduction. However, it did show a significant reduction in cases of non-Hodgkin's lymphoma—about 22 percent.[19]

The differences in the two studies could have been due to study protocol, statistical analysis, or even due to differing treatment of crops in France and England. Because there are so many variables, we need to do more studies. The current studies show us that diet has a role in disease progression. When we eat well, our bodies are more capable of protecting us from disease.

---

18   Julia Baudry, et al, "Association of Frequency of Organic Food Consumption with Cancer Risk," *JAMA Internal Medicine,* October 22, 2018, 178(12): 1597-1606.

19   K. E. Bradbury, "Organic Food Consumption and the Incidence of Cancer in a Large Prospective Study of Women in the United Kingdom," *British Journal of Cancer,* April 29, 2014, 110: 2321-2326.

THE DIRTY DOZEN AND THE CLEAN 15

Organic crops are not genetically modified, and they're not sprayed with conventional agricultural chemicals like Roundup. You may not be able to buy all organic food all the time, but there are some easy guidelines you can follow to reduce the amount of herbicides and pesticides in your food. You can consult the "Dirty Dozen" and the "Clean 15." These lists are updated each year as crops are continually tested for levels of chemical residues.

The Dirty Dozen are the non-organic foods you need to avoid because they have a ton of pesticide residue—you can eat these foods if they're organic. It doesn't matter how much you wash these foods; the chemicals are absorbed into the fruit or vegetable. By avoiding these altogether, you reduce your toxic exposure to these substances.

THE DIRTY DOZEN

As of this writing, the "Dirty Dozen" foods list included:[20]

1. Strawberries
2. Spinach
3. Kale
4. Nectarines
5. Apples
6. Grapes

---

20 "Dirty Dozen," *Environmental Working Group*, 2019.

7. Peaches
8. Cherries
9. Pears
10. Tomatoes
11. Celery
12. Potatoes

The Clean 15 are the foods you don't have to worry about buying organic because they don't have a lot of pesticide exposure to begin with. If you are health-conscious and on a budget, this is something I would recommend.

THE CLEAN 15

As of this writing, these conventionally grown foods had low levels of agricultural chemical residues:[21]

1. Avocados
2. Sweet corn
3. Pineapples
4. Frozen sweet peas
5. Onions
6. Papayas
7. Eggplants
8. Asparagus
9. Kiwi
10. Cabbage

---

21 "Clean 15," *Environmental Working Group*, 2019.

11. Cauliflower

12. Cantaloupe

13. Broccoli

14. Mushrooms

15. Honeydew melon

INFLUENCING YOUR EPIGENETICS

Cancer cells are mutated regular cells. These mutations occur as cells divide and replicate; our genetic code sometimes gets copied improperly in the process. This creates problems as the scrambled code dictates the new cell's processes.

Not all cancers are genetic, however, and there is a secondary mechanism by which cells can become cancerous: through epigenetics, or our gene expression.

MEDICAL CRASH COURSE
DEFINING EPIGENETICS

Before we get into epigenetics, it may be worthwhile to review genes and DNA. Genetics is what makes us who we are; it is the study of inherited characteristics, otherwise known as genes. Genes carry DNA, or instructions, that are inherited from our parents that ultimately determine our individual characteristics, such as eye color or hair color.

As a cell reads the instructions for its various processes in the genetic code, certain genes are turned on and others are turned off. There are hundreds of genes that can be associated with the development of cancer, but they don't necessarily result in cancer for every individual. That's because our cells are constantly being turned on and off by our daily lifestyle practices.

Epigenetics is this mechanism for regulating gene activity that determines which genes are turned off or on. Recent research has shown that modification of gene expression is influenced by lifestyle practices, environmental exposure to toxins, and ongoing infections that create inflammation in our bodies. Lifestyle choices such as nutrition, exercise, quality of sleep, stress management, social contact, and spirituality all have the ability to modulate our gene expression. When our lifestyle practices are optimal, our regulatory gene switch for disease is off. However, when our practices are poor, our regulatory gene switch for disease is turned on.

We refer to these modulating cell processes as *pathways*. These pathways represent chemical responses (in the form of enzymes) that are triggered by epigenetics. A few specific pathways are associated with the onset of cancer. Later in this section we'll take a closer look at the notable ones that can be affected by lifestyle choices: mTOR and AMPK.

Mutations are held in check by a healthy functioning immune system. If your immune system is compromised and in a chronic inflammatory state, your ability to keep those mutations in check is decreased. If you're living a lifestyle that creates chronic inflammation, you're likely to put yourself into a state where you will suffer from a chronic disease, and possibly even cancer.[22]

If we are able to control our gene expression, then we can upregulate the positive gene expressions that fight cancer and downregulate the negative gene expressions that promote cancer. The epigenetic pathways that dictate the processes within our cells are interconnected: when you influence one pathway, you create ripple effects in other pathways. Because of the interconnected nature of these pathways, lifestyle changes have the potential to positively affect multiple pathways at once.

Diet is an easy, yet powerful way of regulating our gene expression. For example, if you eat cruciferous vegetables (e.g., broccoli or Brussels sprouts), it turns off the gene for cancer cell growth by releasing antioxidant and detoxification enzymes that protect against carcinogens: substances that cause cancer. The chemical sulforaphane, found in cruciferous vegetables, is responsible for this action. Keep in mind that studies that demonstrate this use a highly

---

22 "Epigenetics: How It Works and What It Means for Cancer Research," *Dana-Farber Cancer Institute*, 2018.

concentrated form of sulforaphane. It is unclear whether sulforaphane could be used to lower cancer risk or reduce cancer growth, but population studies have linked a higher density intake of cruciferous vegetables with a significantly reduced risk of cancer.[23] This is why it's important to eat a variety of nutritious foods: not only do they have essential antioxidants, vitamins, and minerals, but certain foods also have an effect on our gene expression.

A variety of drugs are used to manage cancer symptoms, but it's nearly impossible for a specific drug to work optimally because the drug does not help with faulty gene expression. Faulty gene expression is due to unhealthy diet, lack of exercise, and toxin exposure. Taking a drug to resolve the resulting epigenetic issues is like slapping a Band-Aid over a deep wound—it's going to keep bleeding if your lifestyle choices are sub-optimal.

No one addresses this when treating cancer. They just engage in symptom management, but that doesn't get to the root of the problem. Recurrences of cancer often happen because people return to their previous lifestyle, whether it includes a high volume of stress, a highly processed diet, or lack of exercise.

We have over 25,000 genes in our bodies, so there are many

23   C. Bosetti, et al, "Cruciferous Vegetables and Cancer Risk In a Network of Case-Controlled Studies," *Annals of Oncology*, 2012, 23(8): 2198-2203.

other genes that can be influenced by lifestyle factors. Specific genes are related to different cancers, so if you've been diagnosed with cancer or want to prevent a specific cancer for which you have a family history, it's important to identify the cancer's related genes so you can effectively alter and modulate your lifestyle to positively regulate gene expression.

With my cancer, non-Hodgkin's lymphoma, the mTOR pathway is a huge ringleader, and it has a direct relationship with the AMPK pathway, so influencing one creates changes in the other. Let's take a closer look at what these two pathways do.

MEDICAL CRASH COURSE
TRACKING ENZYME PATHWAYS

The signaling pathway mTOR (which stands for mammalian target of rapamycin, in case you're curious) is responsible for cell proliferation. Turn on the mTOR pathway, and cells replicate faster. Turn it off, and replication slows down. The mTOR's natural function is meant to help our bodies create new cells, but it can go into overdrive, and then we create too many cells—which creates more opportunity for them to mutate.

The AMPK pathway (which is the acronym for the enzyme AMPK-activated protein kinase) shuts off the mTOR pathway. AMPK is responsible for *autophagy*, the process of destroying and eliminating unneeded cells. Turn up the AMPK, and you turn down mTOR, which prevents cell growth and reduces the likelihood of producing mutated cells.

The AMPK pathway is upregulated through exercise and muscle contraction, proper nutrition from organic foods, eating in time-restricted windows (which I'll talk about in the upcoming section), and sleeping well. All these behaviors help downregulate the mTOR pathway and slow cell proliferation.

But let's say you're a person who exercises well but sleeps poorly—you will still promote the mTOR pathway. It's a delicate balancing act.

In addition to influencing our epigenetics, these lifestyle habits create multiple anti-cancer benefits. Eating well helps reduce blood sugar and increase insulin sensitivity. Getting proper nutrition and sufficient exercise reduces inflammation. With positive lifestyle changes, our entire bodily functions will work more favorably to protect against cancer.

Labs have produced medications that target these pathways, but often we can ingest the same compounds naturally through our foods. For example, the compound quercetin, found in apples, has an effect on one of the other pathways associated with lymphoma. By taking a pill to ingest this one compound, you can influence one particular element of the pathway. Or you can eat apples and other fruits and vegetables to affect a variety of pathways at once: P13K, AKT, and Myc are three more pathways associated with lymphoma that respond to a healthy diet of whole foods.

To provide your body with the optimum opportunity to deactivate cancer-promoting pathways, you need to adopt a variety of positive lifestyle habits. That's why it's important to not only eat healthy foods but also to practice positive behaviors. Exercise is one aspect. Another aspect is positive mood and spirituality. These all promote positive gene expression. One last lifestyle habit related to diet that has a positive effect on these pathways is fasting.

THE BENEFITS OF FASTING

Beyond *what* you eat, *when* you eat is another component of maintaining ketosis and reducing inflammation. Intermittent fasting is an excellent tool to help your body function optimally.

Essentially, intermittent fasting is when you reduce your feeding window. Rather than eating meals spaced out through the entire day, you restrict your mealtimes to an eight- or twelve-hour period. By doing so, you allow your body to get into a state of ketosis between feeding windows. Some of the beneficial effects of fasting kick in with as little as 12 hours and grow more with fasting from 24-48 hours.

Your metabolism is always in gear whenever you're eating, and in the course of a normal day, your body spends its time digesting, eating, or preparing for the next meal. When those feeding windows are long, your metabolism functions around the clock. Your body doesn't have a chance to rest.

When in a fasted state, you achieve what's called *cellular autophagy*, which is the state where the body repairs itself.[24] Specifically, it is the process by which cells degrade and then eliminate or recycle dysfunctional proteins. If allowed to accumulate, these dysfunctional proteins can contribute to poor tissue or organ function or worse, become cancerous. Autophagy allows the body to fight off potential mutations, reducing the chances of acquiring cancer. Studies in mice have shown that mTOR activity is markedly decreased when in a fasted state.[25]

Additional benefits of fasting include improving brain health, slowing the process of aging, improving body composition, and improving cardiovascular health.

I began with intermittent fasting. I would do all my eating during an eight-hour window and then fast for sixteen hours. My last meal would be at 6 p.m., and then my first meal the next day would be at 10 a.m. Whatever I typically ate during

---

24   Robert Chen and Sumeet Sharma, "Intermittent Fasting," *HVMN*, July 10, 2016.

25   Merdad Alirezaei, "Short-Term Fasting Induces Profound Neuronal Autophagy," *Autophagy*, 2010, 6(6): 702-710.

the course of a day would be during that eight-hour period. As I practiced intermittent fasting, my body became more adapted and I was able to tolerate this easily after putting this into practice over several months. I then increased my food restriction slowly until I reached 24 hours and 36 hours of fasting.

Moderation is important in everything. When it comes to my typical fasting weekly schedule, I spend Monday through Friday doing intermittent fasting for sixteen hours a day, and then Saturday is when I go all out. I eat whatever I want—whether it's desserts or pizza—and Sunday is my day to completely fast for twenty-four hours. My last weekend meal is usually Saturday at 6 p.m., and I fast until Sunday at 6 p.m.

Giving your body a little bit of everything in moderation does more for you than specifically doing one modality. Our bodies are adaptive, and if you do something for a long period of time, your body adapts and the benefits aren't as apparent after a while. By mixing it up, you introduce a little bit of confusion, and your body doesn't get accustomed to the same routine. If I were to create an even more optimal schedule, I would probably do a forty-eight-hour or seventy-two-hour fast at quarterly intervals. Fasting greater than 36 hours is best done under medical supervision.

But if you have a regular practice of some sort of fasting, it will be helpful for you. The whole idea is to give your body a break from digestion so it can repair.

EATING WELL ON A BUSY SCHEDULE

When I was trying to have my cancer regress during the watch and wait period, I tried to provide my body with antioxidants and nutrients, and I completely cut out processed food and replaced my diet with all organic foods. I was in a position to do that because I wasn't working at the time. I could spend the necessary time buying and preparing the food. In that aspect it was easy; I was devoted to it and I liked the challenge. After I was in remission and it became a preventative task to stay in remission, it was almost impossible to maintain on a regular basis because life gets in the way.

There are different ways of accomplishing this goal to eat better. There are meal services to which you can subscribe that provide healthy organic meals. They are prepackaged and prepared and you can order seven days' worth of breakfasts, lunches, and dinners. You can also try food prep services where they provide you with all of the ingredients and give you a recipe. Blue Apron and Green Chef are examples of these services. I prefer Green Chef because it's all USDA organic and non-GMO. You get six servings for 90 bucks—if you were to eat out for six meals, you would spend much more than that.

There are times when I want to eat out, and I do so because

it's entertaining, work-related, or because I have a craving. I believe if you eat well 75 percent of the time, that's sufficient.

Chapter Six

THE SCIENCE OF SUPPLEMENTATION

At the time of my diagnosis, I was living in Florida and spending time outside in the sun golfing or playing tennis or hiking. You'd think that my vitamin D levels would be high, as sunlight facilitates the process of converting vitamin D through the skin. Vitamin D is crucial for proper immune function. It aids in the body's chemical reactions and promotes an anti-inflammatory effect, and it's involved with the epigenetics of 10 to 15 percent of our genes. Obviously, it's important to optimize your vitamin D levels.

When you test for vitamin D, the range for a healthy individual is wide, from 20 to 100 nanograms per milliliter of blood. My count was 19.

I was particularly susceptible to getting sick, so I'd always known I didn't have an optimally-functioning immune system. Before my cancer research, I thought it was just something I was born with. My low vitamin D levels explained, at least partially, why my immune system was compromised. My body didn't have what it needed to fight inflammation and disease.

How does a golfer in Florida get a vitamin D deficiency? For one thing, I have dark skin, and high amounts of melanin have a tendency to block some of the benefits of sunlight. When I spent time outside, I would apply sunblock: add that to skin that was already having a hard time absorbing sunlight, and it became impossible to get proper vitamin D from my environment. I required supplementation.

NUTRIENT DEFICIENCIES

We need certain nutrients for the body to function optimally and fight off inflammation. While we're meant to get these nutrients from our diet and environment, we often don't: the standard American diet, which contains heavily processed foods, is lacking in many of the nutrients we need. That's why eating a balanced diet of whole foods is essential. As we discussed in the last chapter, particular nutrients help facilitate specific gene expressions. As the components of our food turn certain pathways on or off, we can promote or reduce inflammation. When our bodies have the right nutrients, they're less likely to develop inflammatory conditions, We can dial in our balance of nutrients with supplementation.

Supplements are agents we can use to promote a healthy gut, create anti-inflammatory effects, and assist in our epigenetic pathways.

MEDICAL CRASH COURSE
TESTING FOR INFLAMMATION

You can get blood work done to understand what shape your immune system is in, and specific markers can indicate whether your body is currently in an inflammatory state. Ask your primary care physician to check the following levels:

- hs-CRP: This is a protein released by the liver and used to assess the presence of inflammation and is generally elevated with tissue destruction, infection, inflammation, or cancer.

- ESR: This is a non-protein reactant that measures the rate of clumping of red blood cells. This is elevated in states of malignancy, connective tissue disease, infections, and other inflammatory diseases.

- Proinflammatory Cytokines: Proteins such as IL-6, TNF-alpha, IL-1b are released by the immune system in response to inflammatory activity

- Vitamin D: This nutrient is necessary for the proper functioning of your immune system, so it's important to know whether you are within normal levels.

It's important to look at all the inflammatory markers together, as each one individually can give you an incomplete picture. Having your healthcare professional review all these levels together will provide a more complete measure of the various stages of your body's inflammatory status. Additionally, if you implement strategies to reduce inflammation, you can test periodically for these markers to gauge the effects of your efforts.

When you get a typical panel of blood work done, blood sugar and insulin tests are standard. You can request additional tests, from your inflammatory markers to tests for gut microbiome diversity, specific levels of vitamins, and even your omega-3 breakdown.

The blood tests required to monitor the nutritional condition of your body are costly, and if you don't have health insurance, they will be out-of-pocket expenses. Knowing your levels can give you an important window into how your systems are doing and what you need in terms of supplementation. Companies such as SpectraCell and Genova Diagnostics offer in-depth laboratory tests for these levels.

In my research, I focused on supplements that could help

me reduce inflammation and support my microbiome. The specific supplements mentioned in this chapter all have the potential to benefit you if your inflammatory markers are high.

Once you've determined which supplements to take, ask your doctor if any of them are offered by prescription. Some supplements are prescription-based and can be covered by health insurance.

After you've taken supplements for a while, it's important to retest your levels so you can determine whether they're effective. You can't assume that the lowest dose will be within a therapeutic range for you. I recommend retesting every three to four weeks to make sure the supplements you're taking are effective. If the levels aren't increasing, you may need to change the brand you're using or increase the dosage.

Not all supplements are created equal. Some supplements have fillers and may even be devoid of the vitamin they're promoting. Rather than shopping for supplements at a GNC or Walmart, I go to stores where there are knowledgeable staff members who can recommend high quality brands.

Each of the supplements below aids in important functions in the body and can be helpful to take if you are fighting cancer or trying to optimize your health and reduce your cancer risk.

VITAMIN D

Vitamin D is a necessary nutrient for a wide range of our body's processes and plays a huge role in our gene expression. Before jumping to supplementation for this important nutrient, you should expose your body to more sunlight. I don't recommend you spend hours in the sun; it's a risk-reward ratio. If you get a sunburn, you're at risk for melanoma and skin cancer. But it will benefit you to get out in the sun a few times a day for short periods. The intensity of the sun is greatest between 11am and 2pm, depending on your geography; you'll get better, direct exposure during those times and will optimize your natural vitamin D levels. Be cautious and apply sunscreen when necessary to prevent sunburn.

If you've determined supplementation is necessary, you can take vitamin D in pills or drops. Pills absorb more slowly, and if you have a poorly functioning GI system, you may not be able to absorb as much. The liquid drops are fat soluble, and they are absorbed more easily and quickly. Whatever you take, it's important to check your levels on a regular basis, to check the effectiveness of your regimen. This must be done in a physician's office by blood draw. Your goal is to maintain a range between 20 and 100ng/ml. Even if you're not presently sick, it's important to know whether your vitamin D levels are within the range to support your immune system.

Two co-factors are needed for vitamin D absorption: magnesium and vitamin K2. If you are in the sun a lot and your levels are low, it could be due to various factors, including having dark skin, applying too much sunblock, or being deficient in foods with magnesium and vitamin K2. Magnesium is found in many green leafy vegetables and in pumpkin seeds. K2 is typically found in hard cheeses. Making sure you get sunlight and a varied diet can help you optimize your body's natural vitamin D level without supplementation. When all else fails, supplementation is the way to go.

MAGNESIUM

The mineral magnesium is used in hundreds of our body's enzyme reactions. On average, most people are deficient in magnesium simply because they are consuming a standard American diet and not ingesting enough vegetables. As noted above, leafy greens are a great source of magnesium.

A very specific test is required to ascertain magnesium levels, called a targeted red blood cell test. This test isn't the first choice for many primary care physicians; many physicians opt for a serum level test. The red blood cell (RBC) test is more expensive, but it is far more accurate. Fifty to 60 percent of your body's magnesium is stored in your bones, and less than 1 percent is usually flowing in the bloodstream, measured by a serum blood test. It's possible to have a low serum level when you're not magnesium deficient, because the magnesium is being effectively absorbed in your bones. Similarly, a high serum level may indicate that your bones are not absorbing magnesium properly. The RBC test looks at levels of magnesium in the red blood cells themselves, which originate in our bone marrow. As a result, the RBC test gives a much more accurate picture of the overall levels of magnesium in your body.[26]

Mild to moderate symptoms of magnesium deficiency include but are not limited to: anxiety, depression, fatigue, insomnia, headaches, muscle cramping, shortness of breath, and cardiac arrhythmia. Our bodies try to be in homeostasis all the time, so if we don't have enough magnesium available in our bloodstream, our bodies will pull magnesium from bones and tissues to restore those levels in the serum. That will leave your bones and soft tissues deficient. If you feel like your muscles are always in knots, that may be a sign of magnesium deficiency.

It's good to take magnesium on a regular basis, but you do need to exercise caution in dosing. Too much magnesium can produce GI side effects like cramping and diarrhea. There are a few different forms of magnesium supplements: magnesium glycinate is a form of magnesium with an amino acid attached, which enhances absorption and controls side effects. Magnesium glycinate also aids people with sleeping, and it doesn't have the side effects that come with other modes of magnesium.

---

26 Thomas DeLauer, "Serum Magnesium vs. RBC Magnesium," *Jigsaw Health,* April 6, 2018.

MELATONIN

Sleep is the most important lifestyle factor to promote healing. It's restorative and turns on many of the reparative pathways in our epigenetics. We need a good amount of sleep, and if we're not getting enough, our body doesn't have a chance to heal and recover.

Melatonin is often used to assist with sleep, and a combination of melatonin and magnesium is a good way to aid in restorative sleep. There's evidence to show that high doses of melatonin can prolong survival for patients suffering certain types of cancers.[27]

Melatonin, overall, has an antioxidant property so it reduces inflammation just by simply taking it on a regular basis. If you want to enhance natural production, getting sunlight is the most effective way as that increases our production of melatonin. You can also consume plant foods such as flax seeds, orange bell peppers, tart cherry juice, walnuts, tomatoes, mustard seeds, gogi berries, almonds, and raspberries to boost levels of melatonin.

OMEGA-3 FISH OIL

Nutritionists have often noted that the typical standard

---

27   Y. M. Wang, et al, "The Efficacy and Safety of Melatonin in Concurrent Chemotherapy or Radiotherapy for Solid Tumors," *Cancer Chemotherapy and Pharmacology*, May 2012, 69(5): 1213-20.

American diet has a disproportionately high ratio of omega-6 fatty acids to omega-3 fatty acids. This abnormally high ratio is pro-inflammatory and ingesting diets that are high in omega-3 can offset the negative effects of inflammation. Diets rich in omega-3 fatty acids can reduce inflammation and oxidative stress and promote anti-aging.

Numerous studies and research have shown supplementation with fish oil or consumption of oily fish lowers blood pressure,[28] reduces triglycerides,[29] prevents primary and secondary cardiovascular disease,[30] and reduces levels of depression.[31] A strong inverse association was observed between consumption of omega-3 fatty acids and risk of non-Hodgkins lymphoma.[32] Omega 3 fatty acids may reduce the risk of breast cancer, but may increase the risk of prostate cancer. In a study of patients in advanced lung cancer, subjects taking omega-3 supplements experienced better out-

---

28 M. C. Morris, F. Sacks, and B. Rosner, "Does Fish Oil Lower Blood Pressure? A Meta-Analysis of Controlled Trials," *Circulation,* August 1993, 88(2): 523-33.

29 J. P. Miller, et al, "Triglyceride Lowering Effect of MaxEPA Fish Lipid Concentrate: A Multicentre Placebo Controlled Double Blind Study," *Clinica Chimica Acta,* 1988, 178(3): 251-9.

30 P.M. Kris-Etherton, W. S. Harris, L. J. Appel, "Fish Consumption, Fish Oil, Omega-3 Fatty Acids, and Cardiovascular Disease," *Circulation,* November 2002, 106(21):2747-57.

31 M. Rondanelli, et al, "Effect of Omega-3 Fatty Acids Supplementation on Depressive Symptoms and on Health-Related Quality of Life in the Treatment of Elderly Women with Depression: A Double-Blind, Placebo-Controlled, Randomized Clinical Trial," *Journal of the American College of Nutrition,* February 2010, 29(1):55-64.

32 Bridget Charbonneau, et al, "Trans Fatty Acid Intake Is Associated with Increased Risk and N3 Fatty Acid Intake with Reduced Risk of Non-Hodgkins Lymphoma," *The Journal of Nutrition,* 2013, vol. 143(5): 672-81.

comes and were able to receive more chemotherapy cycles than subjects not using omega-3s.[33]

Dr. Weil advocates eating fish such as salmon, which has a high amount of omega 3s, as well as sardines and Alaskan black cod. If you're also eating healthy fats such as olive oil, walnuts, and avocados several times a day, you will have optimal levels of omega 3s. But for those who don't consume fish regularly, supplementation can be done with fish oil. I recommend supplementing with fish oil even if you're getting these foods into your diet. Omega-3s tend to be deficient in our regular diets.

You want to get fish oil that is sourced from freshwater fish rather than farmed fish. Farmed fish are typically genetically modified, and their omega-3 content is nonexistent.

I use Nordic Naturals, which sources oil from freshwater fish up in the Nordic areas where high levels of omega 3 have been found.

PROBIOTICS

We want to promote an environment in our gut that has beneficial bacteria, so we don't have a state of dysbiosis. Adding

---

33   R. A. Murphy, et al, "Supplementation with Fish Oil Increases First-Line Chemotherapy Efficacy In Patients with Advanced Non-Small Cell Lung Cancer," *Cancer*, 2011, 117(16):3774-80.

probiotics assists with this goal. We can get probiotics naturally through fermented foods like yogurt, sauerkraut, and kimchi, and through fermented drinks like kombucha.

If you can't get probiotics through food sources, probiotic supplements provide an alternative but can be expensive. Probiotics come in various strains, and you want to rotate your probiotics to increase the diversity of good bacteria in your gut.

Because probiotics are living strains of bacteria, they need support to make it to the gut. Make sure you include a prebiotic—a food that the bacteria can metabolize—with your probiotic. The most effective prebiotic is fiber, which you can get from fruits and vegetables. A diet rich in those should be sufficient to get enough fiber needed to feed the good bacteria.

TURMERIC

Curcumin is the active ingredient in turmeric, and it has been shown to have potent anti-inflammatory effects on the body, as well as anti-cancer effects. A study published in 2016 detailed the mechanisms of action of curcumin on enzyme pathways reducing tumor cell proliferation, inducing apoptosis (cell death) and autophagy, and reducing metastasis.[34]

---

34   A. R. Pavan, et al, "Unraveling the Anticancer Effect of Curcumin and Resveratrol," *Nutrients*, 2016, 8(11): 628.

Turmeric can be added as a spice to normal foods or ingested as a supplement.

To make turmeric more bioavailable, it's important to combine it with fat to act as a carrier, so the body can absorb it without it being eliminated too quickly. Alternately, you can combine turmeric with black pepper, which contains a chemical called piperine that allows the body to absorb curcumin more easily. Doses in clinical settings are 400mg-600mg three times a day.

Taking too much turmeric can lead to gastrointestinal effects like cramping and bloating, so it's important to achieve a balance.

CINNAMON AND BITTER MELON

Cinnamon and bitter melon are helpful in reducing blood sugar because they mimic the effects of insulin. These two compounds increase your uptake of sugar to muscle cells and fat cells, which lowers your blood sugar.

Cinnamon also acts on the P13K pathway—one of the pathways mentioned earlier that are associated with lymphoma. It has shown to have beneficial effects on factors associated with metabolic syndrome, including insulin sensitivity, blood sugar, cholesterol, and body weight. Ultimately, related diseases associated with metabolic syndrome such as stroke, cancer, and Alzheimer's have shown improvement with the usage of this spice.[35] Cinnamon can be taken as a pill supplement, or it can simply be sprinkled on food.

Bitter melon works on the AMPK pathway—the pathway that slows down cell replication and stimulates cellular autophagy and elimination. Bitter melon can be taken in raw form, but it's often so bitter that people find it intolerable. Supplements are available in capsule or pill form. Studies have shown that in addition to its effects of lowering blood sugar, it also has antioxidant activity. Studies in rats have shown this herb can reduce cholesterol and triglycerides.[36]

Both cinnamon and bitter melon are natural herbs, and their side effects are minimal. It's possible, though highly unlikely, to get hypoglycemia from too much ingestion of these substances. These are helpful supplements to upregulate positive gene expression.

COLOSTRUM

Colostrum is a form of milk produced in the mammary glands of mammals. When their offspring consume the colostrum, antibodies (immunoglobulins), prebiotics, pro-

35   Bolin Qin, Kiran S. Panickar, and Richard A. Anderson, "Cinnamon: Potential Role in the Prevention of Insulin Resistance, Metabolic Syndrome, and Type 2 Diabetes," *Journal of Diabetes Science and Technology*, May 2010, 4(3): 685-693.

36   Ashraful Alam, et al, "Beneficial Role of Bitter Melon Supplementation in Obesity and Related Complications in Metabolic Syndrome," *Journal of Lipids*, January 12, 2015.

teins, and other nutrients are passed from the mother to the infant. This is why it's so important to breastfeed: colostrum provides protection against gastrointestinal and respiratory infections and helps support the overall development and function of the human immune system.[37]Additionally, it also establishes beneficial bacteria in the infant's digestive tract.[38]

In non-human studies, research shows that colostrum can restore a leaky gut lining to normal permeability levels. Additionally, animal studies show that colostrum can help repair the injury of the small intestine caused by non-steroidal anti-inflammatory drugs.

Human research is limited, but a study in athletes demonstrated improved immune function with colostrum supplementation. The subjects in the study showed improved resistance to upper respiratory infections when taking colostrum.[39]

Before supplementing with colostrum, I recommend having the blood test drawn to check your immunoglobulins. If your immunoglobulins are low, it's worth trying colostrum for a few months and then rechecking your count. If there is an

37 Lauren H. Ulfman, et al, "Effects of Bovine Immunoglobulins on Immune Function, Allergy and Infection," *Frontiers in Nutrition,* June 22, 2018.

38 M. S. Cilieborg, M. Boye and P. T. Sangild, "Bacterial Colonization and Gut Development in Pre-Term Neonates," *Early Human Development,* 2012, 88(1): 41-49.

39 G. Davison, "Bovine Colostrum and Immune Function After Exercise," *Medicine and Sport Science,* 2012, 59: 62-69.

improvement in the overall count, it's best to continue the supplement. However, if there is no improvement, then you should consider discontinuing. You can adjust the amount as you need or discontinue the supplement if you don't see improved counts.

MEDICAL CRASH COURSE
THE IMPORTANCE OF IMMUNOGLOBULINS

People who have cancer are deficient in immunoglobulins, the antibodies that fight antigens or foreign invaders. Chemotherapy further lowers the body's immunoglobulins. If we don't have enough immunoglobulins, we will constantly be fighting viruses and bacteria and be susceptible to colds and other health issues.

A blood test is used to look at levels of three main immunoglobulins: IgG, IgM, and IgA. If these levels are low, it's an indicator that your immune system needs a boost.

MY RESULTS OF SUPPLEMENTATION

The harsh chemicals used to treat my cancer decreased my immunoglobulins. I began taking colostrum during my chemo treatment, and it seemed to have protective effects on my immune system, despite the toxic chemotherapy chemicals. I was able to travel somewhat and be around people without getting sick.

Two years after my cancer treatment, my immunoglobulin levels still hadn't moved, and my oncologist told me those levels would probably be my new baseline. I didn't accept that; I knew I would be at risk for getting bacterial infections and viruses more easily with a compromised immune system.

I continued taking the colostrum, even though my levels hadn't improved yet. I knew there would be a delay in the response for my counts to improve because my immune system had been so suppressed by the toxic effects of the chemotherapy.

I did everything I could to raise my immunoglobulin count and improve my immunity, including increasing my exercise and my vitamin D supplements. Four years out from my last chemo treatment, my immunoglobulin counts returned to normal.

I believe that a steady intake of colostrum was the biggest factor in increasing my count to what it is today. I now advise anyone with a compromised immune system to take colostrum regularly.

There was a period when I forgot to renew my colostrum supplementation and I missed taking it. Lo and behold, I started getting sick again with colds. My colds would be drawn out, and I got high fevers. I would get bacterial and viral infections all at the same time. I thought, "I can't live my life like this. I need to protect myself better."

And then I remembered that I hadn't been taking colostrum. As soon as I went back on colostrum, I did not get sick as frequently.

There have not been many studies performed on the effectiveness of specific supplements, so it's difficult to show what would be an effective rate or dose for everyone. But you can investigate the effects yourself with qualitative analysis: obtain blood work on a regular basis and see how deficiencies respond to different supplements you try. That's how you'll determine what works for you.

Chapter Seven

RELATIONSHIP LESSONS

During my second month of chemo treatment, my wife and I adopted a second dog. That's when things began to fall apart.

When the third month of treatment was drawing near, my wife's family planned a special ceremony for her grandmother who had passed away a year and a half before. My wife would fly to Alabama for the ceremony and would be away for four days. Two of those days, I was going to be in chemo.

I didn't want her to accompany me to my chemo session. My monthly chemo sessions included a day and a half of infusions. At first, my wife had insisted on coming with me to the sessions. Typically, undergoing chemo is not a painful process. The after-effects are what hit you. I preferred privacy during the sessions because that was a huge, intimate ordeal and I wanted to be alone. We fought a lot about that. She felt I was pushing her away. We didn't understand each other's stances, and there was no bridging that gap.

By the third month of treatment, I had withdrawn myself from everyone. I had stopped reaching out to my brothers, and I was annoyed by my parents, who called constantly about the cancer, always reminding me that I was sick. I craved isolation all the time.

And I was incredibly angry. Anger was the emotion that allowed me to retain functionality from day to day. It allowed me to process what I was going through without being sad and depressed, and I could still be a rock for my wife. Or so I thought.

She asked to go to her grandmother's ceremony, and I knew how important her grandmother had been to her. I told her if it was what she wanted and needed to do, she should go. What was the point of her being with me during the treatment if I was going to refuse her company? I needed help after the treatments, but I wasn't willing to admit it; I could drive and get around still. My wife felt I was pushing her away, and that I didn't want any assistance. She decided to leave on the trip.

I went to my chemo session and brought myself home. Then,

the second dog that we'd just adopted got intense diarrhea. It turned out she'd gotten Giardia, a parasite that causes gastrointestinal distress. I was trying to take care of myself and our two dogs, and it was not a pleasant experience, to say the least. I was completely overwhelmed.

When she came back, we sat down to talk. "Please don't leave me again," I said, "because this was too hard to do, recovering from chemo and taking on all the responsibilities of the house and the dogs by myself." She understood and agreed not to leave again. But the incident had weakened our relationship.

The next month, one of my wife's best friends was moving from Florida to Washington for her husband's military deployment. The friend needed to find a place to live in a short period of time, and she didn't want to find a place by herself. She asked my wife if she would come to Washington and help her find a place.

I had another chemo session coming up. My wife decided to go anyway. She was gone for eight days, and during that time I wasn't getting support from friends. I was on my fourth month of chemo, and the treatments had taken a toll on my body. When my wife got back, things really started going downhill. We got into a huge argument. It wasn't fair, I said—a lot of the household duties were placed on me to complete, and I needed help. I couldn't do everything I did previously. It was clear, in our argument, that we were struggling to communicate. We had grown further and further apart.

She left. She went to stay with her family, and I was left to fend for myself during the rest of my chemo days.

I wasn't sad—I was angry. That's the emotion I had utilized to get through the entire process. The anger allowed me to function—maybe not optimally, but at least I was functioning. I didn't grieve or cry. I was just alone with my anger.

My immunoglobulin counts had dropped so dangerously low by the time my last round of treatment came up that my physicians decided to cancel the sixth round of chemo. They redid the scans as they normally do at the completion of chemo, and everything was normal. The PET scans showed that all the tumors in my body had completely regressed. No remnants of cancer were left. Everything had worked.

Maybe I should have been elated, but instead I was scared. The trouble with chemo is that while it may kill the cancer, it leaves you with a weakened immune system. I was so severely depleted that the simplest cold could kill me. And I had no support network. A few months later, my wife and I divorced.

LEARNING HOW TO LEAN ON PEOPLE

Going through cancer is an intimate process. Many times, people go through cancer treatment without friends and relatives around. Only your immediate household members see you go through this. I think I would have been in a better place mentally and emotionally if I'd had support. I would have benefited from asking my oncologist for a referral to a therapist, grief counselor, or support group, and I think oncologists should be more forthcoming in recommending mental health support to their patients.

When I learned I would have to go through chemo, it was the unknown that was scary because I always had to have control. Going through the process of cancer meant that the next few months would be full of unknowns—whether I would be sick, whether I would be able to do the things I enjoyed, or whether I'd have the family I'd always wanted. Throughout the next eight months, I tried to read and implement everything I learned to better my health and hopefully to change the prognosis if not the severity of the disease.

A support network is important for helping a cancer patient deal with their treatment and their prognosis. In addition to the intense anger I felt at my ill health, I became incredibly withdrawn during treatment, because in my view, the friends I expected to be there for me weren't. I only occasionally saw friends after I was diagnosed, and when they asked how I was, our conversations were superficial. I felt there was no depth to their concern, and I didn't know how to ask them for what I needed—which was to feel normal.

To have people express that they care would've been a nice pick-me-up. I didn't get that, which further fueled my anger. I began to develop a mistrust toward people.

My parents constantly called me, but this felt like more of a nuisance than a help because it reminded me that I was sick. I desperately needed to be around people and not be treated as a sick person.

My parents were understandably hurt. They didn't know how to react. But they didn't ask what I needed, and I pushed them away because I felt they weren't doing me any good. I was left alone. I didn't go out. I had no friends to hang out with or check up on me because I had pushed them all away, and I had no responsibilities or obligations because I wasn't working at the time.

Connection can be difficult for people with cancer because it's taboo to talk about being sick. For me, there was also ego involved: I didn't want people to feel sorry for me. I also found it difficult to talk about my emotions. But unless you convey your emotions to your loved ones, they're not going to know what you need. A particular kind of distance is created when we find it uncomfortable to talk about what's going on; it creates a lack of communication about the sick person's needs. It's important to keep lines of communication open to express desires, needs, and wants.

Had someone asked me, "What do you need?" I would have said, "I just need to escape." I may have needed to talk more about how I was feeling and what I was going through with my cancer—but at the same time, I didn't need to be constantly reminded that I was sick. I needed to be reminded of the bigger picture and my reasons to fight.

I needed to change my maladaptive thinking. It created a vicious cycle: I felt sad, I felt lonely, and I looked for rejection and hostility in my interactions. It was pivotal to flip that around. I needed a sense of optimism.

A few friends from high school and college knew what was going on, and some came down to visit. Those times were great—finally, for a few hours, I felt like I wasn't sick. It was good for the soul. It made me want to fight and live life again. In those moments, I remembered that life is not all that bad.

THE HEALTH EFFECTS OF LONELINESS

To this day, I have not fully recovered from the introversion and distrust of people that grew in that time. I had turned off God in this process because I was so angry. There was no spirituality in my life, and the loneliness was a never-ending downward spiral.

I would later learn the effect this had on my health. Studies have shown that weak social relationships are as much of a risk factor for mortality as smoking and alcohol consumption. It exceeds other risk factors such as physical inactivity and obesity.[40] Social isolation needs to be addressed in people suffering from disease. We're not meant to be alone; we're meant to have the support of other people. Bonds and relationships are important for our well-being, and as these studies show, for our longevity. The lonelier we are as a society, the worse off we are individually.

A 2015 study even found that loneliness has an impact on our gene expression. Those who were lonely had greater states of inflammation and a weaker immune response than those who weren't lonely.[41]

For me, loneliness triggered more anger and put me in a constant state of fight or flight. As a result, I had an overproduction of stress hormones in my body, which exacerbated the inflammatory conditions in my body and further weakened my already compromised immune system.

My body had become fatigued from the chemo, and my BMI was higher than it should have been. I knew this was com-

---

40 Julianne Holt-Lunstad, Timothy B. Smith, and J. Bradley Layton, "Social Relationships and Mortality Risk," *PLOS Medicine*, July 2010.

41 Honor Whiteman, "Loneliness Alters the Immune System to Cause Illness, Study Finds," *Medical News Today*, November 24, 2015.

promising my health. Now that I was in remission, I didn't want a relapse; I needed to improve my physical health and the health of my connections. I was determined to get myself out of the funk I was in.

I was at my lowest point, and I needed a change. "Why not increase the complexity of my life and just move?" I thought. And suddenly, I decided to move from Jacksonville to D.C, where my parents lived, and where I still had connections to college and high school friends.

MOVING ON

Within a year, I had gone through three of the most stressful experiences humans face: I'd gotten sick, gone through a divorce, and made a major move. As I previously mentioned, I'd seen a therapist off and on before my cancer diagnosis, just to check in emotionally, but she had passed away, and I hadn't sought out another therapist. That lack of support exacerbated the stress of these major life events.

But after my move, things began to change for the better. I reconnected with Adam, the trainer I'd worked with before my cancer. I began to train with him three to four times per week, and we reformulated a bond. I began to get back into physical shape, and I was able to reconnect with Adam as a friend.

I began to realize that the ways I'd alienated myself from

people had made a negative impact on me. I took the initiative and reached out to people. I realized that my ego had gotten in the way of reaching out; I'd been expecting people to call me because of what I'd been through. But if anybody was going to resurrect and reform relationships, I had to do it. I learned that people were genuinely concerned for my well-being. Some people hadn't stayed in contact with me because life just got in the way, as it often does.

Moving to DC meant leaving my whole history with cancer and my divorce behind. It was, in essence, a way of being reborn. Once that was behind me, I no longer harbored the anger that had been plaguing me for all those months. Although I still had a sense of mistrust toward people in general, I did trust my family and long-time friends and maintained those relationships.

Bonding with new people was difficult because I had learned to be introverted, and I thought I had become content with being alone. I'm still working on that. It's a special challenge for me because I don't go into an office on a daily basis, I'm no longer married, and I'm older, so it's harder to form bonds with others who are busy with families and obligations.

During this time, I got accepted into my fellowship in integrated medicine at University of Arizona, directed by Dr. Andrew Weil. I was encouraged; it was a very competitive program, and I had been certain I had no chance of getting in. As I began to read and study, I integrated everything I was learning into my lifestyle. The program gave me a blueprint for how to live my life—the blueprint I've relayed in this book. I began to reconnect not only with my health but with my spirituality. I returned to a meditation practice, which I'd had in the past but had abandoned throughout my cancer journey.

A new purpose sparked within me: I realized there was a reason behind my cancer and my survival. There was a reason the cancer hadn't killed me, a reason I'd reconnected with Adam and recovered my physical strength and my relationships. There was a reason I'd gotten into the field of integrative medicine. If I wasn't supposed to beat cancer, those elements wouldn't have appeared in my life. This perspective fueled a new, optimistic sense of well-being.

I came to believe that if you project negative energy, the universe responds by sending negative energy back. When you project positive energy, the universe responds by giving you positive energy. There is literature to support that positivity and optimism are good for our overall health and well-being, and as I began to tap into my own positive outlook, it became a spiritual guideline that I followed as I rebuilt my life in remission.

MEDICAL CRASH COURSE
TENDING TO YOUR MENTAL HEALTH

The mental aspect of a cancer journey has as much impact on your overall well-being as your physical health. I navigated my journey alone, and I have no doubt that if I had connected to support from friends, family, and a therapist earlier, I would have experienced better outcomes. A few simple guidelines can help you tap into your relationships for support.

1. Find a therapist or support group. You need guidance and expertise to navigate this ordeal of cancer. I didn't have anyone in my life pushing me to seek counseling, and if I did, I probably would have resisted it. But it should be the first thing you seek out to help you deal with the mental and emotional impacts of a cancer diagnosis. Your primary care doctor or oncologist can give you a referral.

2. Enhance your social network. Reach out to friends, family, and loved ones. Be willing to communicate your needs and be open about what you're going through.

3. Cultivate a positive outlook. Look for ways to fuel your optimism. When you connect to your purpose, you can begin to focus on a fulfilling life beyond cancer.

Chapter Eight

THE FIGHT'S OVER... NOW WHAT?

Cancer staging varies depending on the type of cancer, but generally speaking, stage IV cancer means that the cancer is advanced and has spread to other parts of the body, or metastasized.

After my last round of chemo, my oncologist performed scans and tests to see if the cancer had shown signs of regression. He also wanted to confirm whether there was any evidence of cancer in my bones; to check that, he needed to perform a bone marrow biopsy.

Bone marrow biopsies are invasive and traumatic procedures.

The procedure involves the doctor inserting a long needle into the hip bone to aspirate blood, bone, and bone marrow. This is typically done while the patient is awake. Once the samples are taken, they are further screened by a pathologist to determine whether there are any abnormalities present. On occasion, the trauma induced by the procedure can have an impact on the body's immune system. Since my immune system was weakened by five toxic rounds of chemotherapy, I was susceptible to any viral or bacterial infection.

I ended up contracting shingles, post bone marrow biopsy— an experience so painful I wouldn't wish it on my worst enemy.

Shingles is a viral infection that causes a painful burning rash on the body. It's caused by the same virus that causes chicken pox. It presents on one side of the body and usually appears on the trunk. In my case, the painful blisters had spread across the left side of my chest and were quite unbearable. Typically, shingles last for one or two weeks, and then the blisters go away. For me, after the blistery rash subsided, I developed postherpetic neuralgia, a complication of shingles that affects the nerves. I had this sharp, burning, lancinating pain on my skin for close to four months. It was so bad that the slightest touch of my shirt against my skin, where the rash had previously been, caused me to have excruciating pain. It was unlike any other pain I've ever felt.

The thing that got me through was that by this time, Adam

and I were training together. The feel-good hormones of exercise were running through my body and making the process of dealing with the pain easier.

Through boxing training, I was releasing all the animosity that had built up over the course of my cancer diagnosis and treatment. Not only was it a good release for exercise purposes, but it became a symbolic release: I could beat up on cancer and all of the negative experiences I had just gone through.

During chemotherapy, I had taken to wearing loose, comfortable clothing. Though I saw myself naked in the mirror every day, I didn't see the slow, incremental physical changes that were happening as I gained weight in my midsection. I could see the changes easily in pictures; in snapshots from one month to the next, the changes were dramatic. My muscle mass had nearly disappeared. Chemo had depleted my energy so much that I was incredibly fatigued by walking short distances. Physical exertion left me out of breath. At that time, my reflection in the mirror reinforced my negative associations with everything: I felt bad, and I looked bad. Because I looked bad, I continued to feel bad, and I didn't want to do anything with my body. It was a perpetual cycle.

As time progressed and chemo became a more and more distant memory, I slowly started to regain some energy. My tolerance for activity increased. I could walk to my mailbox without feeling short of breath. My body began to change, and I built back muscle. This was encouraging and a positive reinforcement for me, reassuring me that cancer was indeed behind me.

The more positive change I saw, the more optimism and positive energy I felt. Cancer didn't define me anymore.

THE EMOTIONAL EFFECTS OF EXERCISE

People who go through cancer are pumped full of drugs that fill their body with toxins. To counteract those effects, it's important to produce feel-good hormones, and you can do this through exercise. When people go through cancer, there's often a feeling of hopelessness that stems from having so much of your health and your life outside of your control. You give your life over to the hands of the doctors. You take the medicines they give you, and you hope your health will change for the better. Exercise is extremely helpful and important because it can give you a sense of well-being and a sense of control. You can't control how cancer treatments will make you feel, but you *can* control the release of endorphins. Exercise-induced release of endorphins helps boost physical health and positive emotions and feelings.

It can take time to see the benefits of exercise. It may not be easy to start physical activity, and you may not perceive the feel-good hormones at first. It takes time for the body to build up your capabilities and reap the benefits.

The problem with medicine today is that it's a practice of treating symptoms. It doesn't hone in on the root cause of the problem. When your body is full of toxins, the natural course of allopathic medicine currently is to give you another medication to combat the toxins you've been exposed to through chemotherapy. Exercise is a natural way to achieve the goal of ridding the body of toxins and replacing them with feel-good hormones.

There are times when medications are useful and life-saving, but it's best to see if you can utilize natural means instead of synthetic means of boosting endorphins, for the same reasons we saw for changing diet: a medication can have an effect on a single element or symptom, but a lifestyle change can activate multiple pathways and create a cascade of benefits in our epigenetics.

During the toxic process of chemo, you want your body to move. If you're sluggish and not getting the blood circulating, you're not able to perfuse the organs and move toxins out of your system. In this way, exercise has two-fold benefits. It helps to flush out toxins, and it boosts substances that improve your mood and well-being.

It's important to be mindful of what you can tolerate. During chemotherapy treatment, just walking was difficult to do, but I wish I had walked more. It would have helped me combat the negative effects of a sedentary lifestyle, and after I looked into the research, I realized it could have had a beneficial effect on my mental health.

MEDICAL CRASH COURSE
BOOSTING YOUR BRAIN CHEMISTRY

Exercise releases a suite of chemicals in your brain that have a positive effect on your mental capacity and mood: serotonin, norepinephrine, BDNF, dopamine, and endorphins.[42]

- **Serotonin** is a neurotransmitter that's pivotal for positively influencing your mood. Depression is characterized by low levels of serotonin, and in some studies, exercise has been shown to be as effective as prescription antidepressants for lifting mood.

- **Norepinephrine** is both a hormone and a neurotransmitter, and it helps us feel more alert and focused. It also assists with memory recall.

- **BDNF** stands for brain-derived neurotrophic factor. It's a growth factor that promotes *neuroplasticity*, which is

---

42   Cathe Friedrich, "5 Brain-Boosting Chemicals Released During Exercise," *Cathe.com*, March 23, 2019.

growth of the brain and its connections. It aids in repair by promoting new formations and repairing damaged cells.

- **Dopamine** is a neurotransmitter that connects to our sense of motivation; it's also the chemical that makes us feel good when we get a reward.

- **Endorphins** are hormones that help us feel less pain and fewer negative side effects from stress.

Interestingly, a low level of serotonin in your brain not only lowers your mood but also lowers your motivation to continue exercising. It's a sort of catch-22. If you don't exercise, you decrease your motivation to exercise. You have to dig deep to go through the motions of exercise to increase the serotonin levels. That in itself will give you the motivation to do more exercise.

Then when you start to see the benefits of the exercise, you will look and feel better and you won't want to waste the momentum you've got going. You will want to maintain the progress you've made.

People are familiar with the "runner's high," which comes from the surge of endorphins that we get through exercise. You don't have to be a runner to get the high: simple exercise such as walking done on a regular basis will produce more of these feel-good chemicals.

BRIDGING THE GAP

When your body is in a state of disease, it can feel incredibly hard to get up off the couch when in fact, that's the thing that will start a positive cycle of motivation. There can be a gap between how one feels when starting an exercise program versus what they actually need to do.

This gap can come with two extremes: on one extreme is the person who isn't doing anything. They're stuck on the couch, and it's a huge effort to begin moving their body. On the other extreme is the person who thinks, "If exercise is beneficial, I'm going to do as much as I can," and they jump straight into training for a marathon. People who over-exercise are actually promoting the mTOR pathway—the pathway that increases cell proliferation. In healthy bodies, too much cell proliferation increases the likelihood of mutations which, if left unchecked, can transform into malignant cells. In bodies burdened with cancer, cell proliferation should be halted, to reduce the spread and growth of the cancer. Also, over-exercise can compromise the gut. Elite athletes often experience physical and emotional stress due to high training demands. This stress can all be attributed to alterations in the gut microbiome that can eventually cause leaky gut syndrome.[43]

---

43   Allison Clark and Núria Mach, "Exercise-Induced Stress Behavior, Gut-Microbiota-Brain Axis and Diet: A Systematic Review for Athletes." *Journal of the International Society of Sports Nutrition*, 2016, 13(43).

My recommendation is conservative. You can get a prescription from your physician to see a physical therapist, who can work you up to a capacity where you should be. They can even help you establish a baseline capacity before you begin chemo. You will then have a benchmark for your post-chemo goals as you return to your normal or even increased fitness level.

READY, GET SET, START

It's helpful to set up an "exercise prescription." Begin by identifying what you're physically capable of doing at the start. Day one of your return to exercise may be defined by extreme difficulty. Perhaps it's difficult enough just to walk out your front door to the mailbox. Take that distance and cut it in half, or otherwise break it down to an amount that doesn't leave you exhausted. Use that as your foundation and build on it gradually.

The next day, you may be able to take just a few steps further. The period of time right after chemo, when you're still feeling depleted and exhausted, is not a time to think about weight training. You can't go wrong with walking. There are so many benefits to walking, including improvements to blood circulation, elimination of toxins, and exposure to sunshine and the outdoors. You get the benefits of vitamin D conversion, and being out in nature instead of cooped up in a hospital room or your living room is empowering and uplifting. If you're able to, do walk with a family member or friend, they can encourage you and give you the positive reinforcement you need; it can be an even more positive experience that benefits your relationships.

Especially if you're returning to exercise after chemo, the point is to slowly build up your capacity, so that you don't end your activity winded, tired, and discouraged. Your exhaustion is not "you"—it's your reaction to the chemo chemicals that are being pumped into your system.

Recognize that how you feel will wax and wane on a daily basis, and even within a 24-hour period. It's important to realize there may be times when you feel dejected over not being able to do what you are normally accustomed to doing. Don't get discouraged; your performance in this time is not a reflection of your innate capacity. It's your body's resistance to the toxicity that's present.

When you can put that in perspective, you can also prevent a discouraged, negative mindset. Rather than fueling negative emotions associated with your capacity and progress, use your exercise to boost your feel-good chemicals, build your aerobic capacity, keep attention on the big picture, and celebrate your progress one step at a time. Little by little, your stamina and endurance will increase.

Walking is typically sufficient during the whole process of

cancer treatment. When you achieve remission or begin to feel better, you can graduate to light strength training or other more vigorous activities, depending on how you feel. A physical therapist can be incredibly helpful to create an exercise plan for you, because they're trained healthcare providers that understand how the body operates in the setting of cancer. They know the limitations that cancer patients typically deal with, and they can help set an appropriate pace for progress. They can prescribe home exercises, and adjust as you gradually improve week by week, until you're either back where you were before you started treatment—or you've exceeded your previous capacity.

When you're cleared by your physician and your physical therapist to resume normal activity, you may want to seek out a personal trainer at a gym to help you increase your capacity.

When I restarted a physical exercise program with Adam, I was at my worst. I felt terrible, and I knew I needed to get back in shape. I knew it would stretch me out of my comfort zone, but it was so important to me to get in shape. I wanted to look good, feel good, and begin to get out and reintegrate with society.

Once I began exercising, I got all those benefits—and so much more. My physical and mental health improved, and I began to repair my connections to others, and ultimately, to myself.

Chapter Nine

SPIRITUAL AFTERCARE

After I had recovered my physical and mental health and begun building my connections and relationships, the last element of my life that needed healing was my relationship with God.

I said before that when I learned I would have to go through chemo, I was angry with God. The reality, though, is that I was angry with anything I *could* be angry with. I couldn't deal with the reality of my diagnosis, and I shut down completely—I shut down mentally, I shut down with my family and friends, and I shut down my relationship with God.

On one particular visit to my folks while I was going through treatment, they suggested I needed to go to the temple with my family to pray. This wasn't an unusual thing; my family is extremely religious and spiritual. They often go to the temple on their own, participate in religious activities, and observe religious holidays.

I never fully espoused our religion, but that doesn't mean I wasn't spiritual. I was reluctant to go to temple and practice my parents' religion when I was younger, because I felt like I was being forced to do it by my parents. Additionally, when I was younger, I was often teased for my Indian heritage, and it had a negative impact on my willingness to practice or acknowledge my family's religion. I rebelled, and my rebellious mentality stuck through adulthood.

When I was diagnosed with cancer, it reinforced my non-spiritual mindset. "Well, if I had practiced religion," I thought, "it still wouldn't have changed anything; I would have ended up with this diagnosis anyway. Screw it—I'm not going to temple. I'm going to be angry." That anger became my necessary fuel to survive.

It was only after a few years had passed in remission that I was finally able to start letting go of that anger and hostility. Maybe I was tired of being angry. I needed to move on and promote positivity if I was going to be healthy and experience a true sense of well-being in my life.

I realized that the essence of living is a balance between the mind, heart, and spirit, and I was disconnected from my heart. I could feel a piece was missing. I was working hard on my physical well-being—eating well, taking supplements, and exercising—but I was neglecting two elements of my health: my emotional and spiritual well-being. I didn't necessarily need to practice religion, but I did need to invoke God back into my life. I felt that connecting to God would help me heal further.

As I would learn, experimenting in the realm of spirituality and trying to balance the mind, body, and spirit takes time. In a society where we seek immediate gratification, patience and persistence can be hard to come by. Changes don't occur overnight but take months and years—and I was just beginning on a journey that is still unfolding.

My first step was to have a talk with God in my head. I had always felt like whenever I would talk to myself, I was really having a conversation with God. I had neglected that practice for a long time, but as I healed, I returned to my meditation practice and began to connect with my spirituality again. I felt that meditation would ground me and get me back into a sense of living more presently and not worrying about the future or reflecting on the past.

THE SCIENCE OF SPIRITUALITY

Research examining the physical, mental, and social health of cancer patients showed that spirituality had a positive effect on all three areas. A large meta-analysis showed that people who were dealing with cancer and maintained spiritual practices reported better physical health and recovery, lowered levels of anxiety and depression, and an increased ability to cope.[44] Specific religious behaviors, such as attending church, didn't matter—it was the patients' overall positive spiritual belief that allowed them to experience better physical and mental health throughout their cancer. If they were disconnected with God, they experienced greater distress and poorer emotional well-being.

A second study showed that *positive* spiritual belief was important. People with a variety of health conditions were studied, from brain and spinal cord injury to stroke and cancer. Participants who held *negative* spiritual beliefs, such as a belief in punishment from a higher power, experienced worse pain and mental and physical health than those who held *positive* spiritual beliefs.[45] Even participants who held a mix of positive and negative spiritual beliefs experienced worse health outcomes than those with positive beliefs.

More studies are needed to safely conclude that spirituality has a positive correlation in fighting cancer and leading to a

---

44   John M. Salsman, et al, "A Meta-Analytic Approach to Examining the Correlation between Religion/Spirituality and Mental Health in Cancer," *Cancer*, August 10, 2015.

45   Angela Jones, et al, "Relationships between Negative Spiritual Beliefs and Health Outcomes for Individuals with Heterogeneous Medical Conditions," *Journal of Spirituality in Mental Health*, April 28, 2015, 17(2): 135-152.

positive outcome, but as I looked into this research, I came to understand the power of mindset. One negative thought can affect your outcome for the worse. Conversely, the more positive your frame of mind, the better your experience will be. Cultivating positivity is a spiritual practice.

I define spirituality as reducing self-centeredness and feeling more connected with the universe. Being religious is one way of being spiritual; having a sense that there is a God enables you to feel connected to a higher power. You can be spiritual without being religious; the core of spirituality is in connecting with the universe that is larger than your individual sense of self.

THE HEALTH EFFECTS OF MINDFULNESS PRACTICE

Mindfulness was the first practice I turned to as I reconnected with my spirituality. Mindfulness is defined as a non-judgmental moment-to-moment awareness. It can be practiced by focusing your attention on an object or the breath or your body or thoughts. Focusing on one particular element allows you to keep your attention on the present and not be chased by memories of the past or anxiety for the future.

It's essential to maintain a positive mindset during the whole process of cancer or any health crisis. The more positive your frame of mind, the better the outcome will be. Negative thoughts can pile onto each other and become a downward spiral, and mindfulness can be a helpful practice to counter that process. When you focus on the present moment, you're not dwelling on negative issues. As you become more practiced with mindfulness, those negative moments will occur less.

Research shows that mindfulness improves stress, anxiety, and depression.[46] It also helps in battling addictions[47] and reducing the emotional components that exacerbate chronic pain.[48] Mindfulness also reduces your fight-or-flight response and physical manifestations of stress, including blood pressure and stress hormone release. With stress reduction comes reduced rumination, increased focus, improved memory, and less emotional reactivity.

A study even determined that mindfulness practice can help people who are exhausted from stress and lack of sleep. In a survey of entrepreneurs, researchers found that those who slept more or engaged in regular mindfulness practices

---

46 "The Evidence," *The Center for Mindfulness Studies*, accessed May 1, 2019.

47 K. Witkiewitz, M. Lustyk, and S. Bowen, "Re-Training the Addicted Brain: A Review of Hypothesized Neurobiological Mechanisms of Mindfulness-Based Relapse Prevention," *Psychology of Addictive Behavior*, July 9, 2012, 27(2): 351-365.

48 Rajguru Parth, et al, "Use of Mindfulness Meditation in the Management of Chronic Pain: A Systematic Review of Randomized Controlled Trials," *American Journal of Lifestyle Medicine*, February 21, 2014.

reported lower levels of exhaustion.[49] Exhaustion is commonplace for entrepreneurs—I certainly experienced it as I ran my business—and mindfulness assists with that problem. It doesn't replace the need for sleep, but it alleviates the stress and resulting exhaustion.

In the beginning, it can be difficult to see progress on a day-to-day basis. (Think of monks who, despite years of practice, are still constantly working on the hard task of staying in the moment.) Our brains are cluttered with so much judgment and thoughts of the future and the past that we're not able to connect in the moment with people. Being mindful helps to reduce judgments, stereotypes, and biases and be present with what is.

BASIC MINDFUL BREATHING

Simply paying attention to your breath is a very easy way to access a state of mindfulness. Breathing is the only function we can perform both unconsciously and consciously; it can be completely involuntary, or completely voluntary. Because of this, we can create powerful effects by learning how to control it.

When we're stressed, our breathing becomes shallow and rapid, and our heart rate accelerates. Deep breaths activate

---

49 Oregon State University, "Mindfulness and Sleep Can Reduce Exhaustion in Entrepreneurs," *ScienceDaily*, February 4, 2019.

the *parasympathetic nervous system*, which governs relaxation and repair. Your heart rate slows, and anxiety and stress are reduced.

When I feel my anxiety and stress levels are high, literally taking a minute or two to breathe deeply is very effective. Many people are used to breathing shallowly, and it takes practice to learn to breathe using your diaphragm. When you take full, deep breaths in and out, you use a lot of muscles that aren't normally utilized. You get much more oxygen into your blood, and you're able to eliminate more toxins. Because breath work enables the parasympathetic nervous system, it reduces our fight-or-flight response and calms the body.

I learned a powerful technique from my program director, Dr. Andrew Weil. He teaches an exercise called 4-7-8.[50] The numbers each correspond to a specific action. You take a deep breath for four seconds, hold it for seven seconds, and exhale for eight seconds. You repeat the cycle four times. He advocates doing it twice a day. Practiced twice a day over a period of weeks or months, this exercise has been shown to reduce blood pressure and heart rate. Dr. Weil has described how doing this breath work exercise helped people with an irregular heart rate return to a regular rhythm. By training you to take deeper breaths, this practice promotes relaxation and counteracts stress hormones that are produced when we're in survival mode.

---

50   Andrew Weil, "How to Perform the 4-7-8 Breathing Exercise," *YouTube*, May 23, 2014.

MODALITIES FOR PRACTICING MINDFULNESS

I was first exposed to meditation when I was in residency around 2003. I practiced transcendental meditation, which is a specific type of meditation in which you're given a personalized mantra by a teacher. You sit in a comfortable position and recite this mantra to yourself, for twenty minutes. Many people are under the impression that you have to clear your mind and let it be blank for "successful" meditation, but that's not the case. Transcendental meditation uses a mantra to center your mind as thoughts come and go.

Guided meditation apps can provide an easy way to begin a mindfulness practice for the first time. There are many options available for download. I like Head Space, a free app that offers guided meditations with an option to pay a subscription for additional practices and techniques.

There are a lot of modalities outside of seated meditation available for a person to practice mindfulness. It's important to have a guide to help you reinforce positive behaviors and mindset. It's not uncommon to have a negative thought come up in your mind, and then beat yourself up over it; that cycle can negatively influence your thought process and outlook. For that reason, it's helpful to practice with a guide or a teacher. A guide can help bring you back to observing the moment and promoting positive well-being.

Therapist-Supported Mindfulness Practices

Many styles of therapy involve mind-body practices and working with a therapist or practitioner in these modalities can deepen your spiritual exploration.

Hypnosis is one modality that helps people focus their intention inward. This can be aided by visualization and imagery. A trained therapist helps encourage inward reflection over outward attention.

Music therapy is used to help people with anxiety, depression, mood disorders, and even chronic pain to manage symptoms and promote relaxation.

Massage therapy and acupuncture can also promote relaxation and offer symptom relief for people undergoing cancer treatment. Massage is often recommended by oncologists to alleviate depression and mood disorders.[51]

Movement-Based Mindfulness

Some mindfulness or spiritual practices incorporate movement to develop mind-body awareness. Yoga combines breathing techniques, physical movement, and meditation to promote health and relaxation. There are a variety of styles you can explore; I do Kundalini yoga, which is a type of yoga that helps move energy through the different chakras

---

51 "About Mind-Body Therapies," *Memorial Sloan Kettering Cancer Center*, 2019.

or energy centers of your body. I feel the energy movement throughout my body, and it helps me focus and become more mindful.

Qi Gong and Tai Chi are two more mind-body practices that help people connect with their spirituality through conscious movement, breathing techniques, and moment-to-moment mindfulness.

Selflessness as a Mindfulness Practice

Another way we can begin connecting to our spirituality is to connect with others in selfless service. A selfless act could be something as simple as listening to a friend or as organized as donating your time to volunteer at a charity. When we assist others in fulfilling their needs, we connect to a purpose greater than ourselves.

As we provide empathy for others, we also connect to our own self-love. When you love yourself, that gets conveyed in the way you are with others.

As I developed my own spiritual practices, I looked for ways to deepen my sense of self-love. For me, the most powerful method to connect with myself—and ultimately, to understand better how to be of service to others—was by exploring psychedelic therapies.

THE POWER OF PSYCHEDELICS

I was drawn to explore psychedelics because of the stories I'd heard from people who had profound, life-changing, and positive experiences. The possibility of using psychedelics to aid in PTSD, depression, and anxiety is being explored more and more by the scientific community; in fact, a 2016 study explored the effects of psychedelics on cancer patients who had been given a life-threatening diagnosis and were suffering from anxiety and depression. Participants were given both low and high doses of psilocybin, and 80 percent of them showed clinically significant decreases in depressed mood and anxiety. They also reported improvements in their mood, relationships, spirituality, and outlook on life.[52]

After my personal trauma of cancer, divorce, and disconnection from people, I wanted to find a therapy that could help me reconnect to myself and to others. Psychedelics seemed like a great place to begin.

In general, I'm a skeptical person, and I look for results. Over the course of ten months of psychedelic therapies, I saw deep-level changes, little by little. My brain chemistry shifted; I no longer get stuck in the whirlwind of self-pity and negative self-worth. Combined with my meditation and

52 Roland R. Griffiths, et al, "Psilocybin Produces Substantial and Sustained Decreases in Depression and Anxiety in Patients with Life-Threatening Cancer," *Journal of Psychopharmacology*, December 30, 2016, 30(12): 1181-1197.

yoga practices to integrate these experiences, I feel a much deeper connection to the universe and to other people.

No prescribed path will work for every individual. What I hope to relay with my experiences is the way this particular path affected me. From my first experience with psychedelics, I began to open an important door to help me trust people again.

SET AND SETTING

The trees were so green and the sky was so bright as I drove home on a road I had traversed hundreds of times. I saw buildings on the side of the road that I had never looked at before. I took notice of the various designs of the numerous homes I was passing. Why didn't I notice this before? It's as if I was driving on this road for the very first time. Additionally, I felt burdenless; I felt lighter and my mind was blank. This was the very first time, in as long as I could remember, that my mind wasn't ruminating. I wasn't thinking of the future, or the past, I was just focused on the present. This was the experience I had coming home after my first underground psychedelic experience.

It was almost as if my brain had slowed down from 100 mph to a nice cruise speed of 45 mph. Rumination is defined as "a mode of responding to distress that involves repetitively and passively focusing on symptoms of distress and on the possible causes and consequences of these symptoms."[53] Evidence now suggests that rumination is associated with psychopathologies including depression, anxiety, binge eating, binge drinking, and self-harm.[54]

The area of the brain where these processes occur is collectively known as the default-mode network (DMN). The DMN also houses the construct we call self or ego. To put this in a more relatable perspective, this area lights up when a Facebook user receives a lot of likes for a post. Under the influence of psilocybin, otherwise known as magic mushrooms, there is reduced activity in the DMN due to reduced blood flow during acute exposure.[55] Interestingly, this quieting of the DMN is also seen in folks who are expert meditators. The lasting effects of psilocybin can vary and it is proposed that the psilocybin functions as a "reset mechanism" for the brain turning the DMN off and back on again, directly improving symptoms of depression.[56]

As I write this, I've had under a dozen or so psychedelic experiences. Each one is different. As I've navigated each

53 Berman, Marc G. et al, "Depression, Rumination and the Default Network," *Social Cognitive and Affective Neuroscience*, 2011, 6(5): 548-555.

54 S. Nolen-Hoeksema, B. E. Wisco, and S. Lyubomirsky, "Rethining Rumination," *Perspectives in Psychological Science*, 2008, 3(5): 400-424.

55 Robin L. Carhart-Harris, et al, "Neural Correlates of the Psychedelic State as Determined by fMRI Studies with Psilocybin, *Proceedings of the National Academy of Sciences of the United States of America*, 2012, 109(6): 2138-43.

56 Robin L. Carhart-Harris, "Psilocybin for Treatment-Resistant Depression: fMRI-Measured Brain Mechanisms," *Scientific Reports*, 2017.

experience, I can conclusively say that "set and setting" is of utmost importance. Timothy Leary describes this in his book *The Psychedelic Experience: A Manual Based on the Tibetan Book of the Dead*, "set" is the mindset or expectation one brings to the experience, and "setting" is the environment in which it takes place.[57] I found out the hard way how important these two facets are in influencing an experience. Some of my worst experiences occurred when I didn't feel safe or when I was in a group setting not knowing anyone. I also felt unsafe in one instance when I didn't know the person conducting the ceremony.

These poor experiences manifested because I went into the experience with anxiety, uncertainty, and a feeling of mistrust. These emotions were magnified during my psychedelic journey and were obviously unpleasant. Even though I had a suboptimal experience, the benefits of the medicine on my brain chemistry still took place. Rumination slowed, and my depressive symptoms decreased.

THE CEREMONY

In my first experience, I signed up for a retreat in psychedelics without having read anything ahead of time; I just trusted the friends who recommended it to me. The facilitator had been conducting ceremonies with psychedelics for over twenty years. We were to be exposed to two medicines,

---

57   Timothy Leary, *The Psychedelic Experience*, New York: Citadel, 2017.

each lasting anywhere from four to six hours, and we would sleep at the retreat space and have an integration session the next morning to discuss our experiences.

The first medicine used was a 3,4-methylenedioxymethamph etamine (MDMA) analog, which is also the active ingredient in ecstasy. I was a little worried about how that would affect my brain, but the doses given were not the same as those in recreational use. Additionally, the medicine was a pure form of MDMA, not something obtained off the streets. MDMA is nicknamed the "heart opener," leaving you more open to people, to interaction, and the experience of the psychedelic that would come next. Before its prohibition in 1985, psycho-therapists were using MDMA as an adjunct to psychotherapy. Under MDMA, there is a significant reduction of metabolism in the brain's amygdala, a region shown to be involved in maintaining the "fear network" of the brain. Additionally, there are elevations in levels of the hormone oxytocin and the neurotransmitter serotonin. This increase translates into an increase in trust and bonding toward others and reductions in anxiety and fear.[58]

I didn't feel much of an effect from the MDMA, at first. As time passed, I was more talkative, a little less anxious, and feeling pretty relaxed. MDMA was definitely kicking in.

---

58 S. B. Thal and M. Lommen, Thal, "Current Perspective on MDMA-Assisted Psychotherapy for Posttraumatic Stress Disorder," *Journal of Contemporary Psychotherapy*, 2018, 48(2): 99–108.

An hour and a half after the dose of MDMA, we were given the second medicine of the ceremony: psilocybin. Within another half hour, everything felt unsteady. I was seeing double and triple; the floor was moving up and down. I went to the bathroom, thinking I would be sick. Psilocybin can often reduce one's ego and in some extreme cases can dissolve the ego and create a sense of oneness with the universe. I felt a terrible sense of fear because I was beginning to understand how strong my ego was, and how difficult it was to relinquish control and simply let go.

People often describe having amazing visuals and images on psilocybin. Mine were dark: I had a visual of falling down a tunnel, trying to grasp at anything to get my bearings. I saw another vision of a curtain in front of me, blocking my view of the world, and for what felt like hours, I went through the motions of trying to look behind the curtain, and not succeeding.

After the experience, I slept for three or four hours, and when I woke up, I felt no stress. This was atypical of me. Usually if I know I'm not going to get enough sleep, I experience intense anxiety, wondering how I will react in front of people and whether I will be able to function without enough sleep. Generally, I have nagging thoughts in my mind about whether people will be judging me. I carry stress in my shoulders, and they tend to feel extremely tight.

But when I woke up after the ceremony, none of those sensations were there. It was as if a huge weight had been lifted off my shoulders. I felt so light. I started to feel an openness and intimate connection with everybody. I felt like they were all my friends. And I was curious—why hadn't I felt that way the night before?

We began our integration discussion, which was an opportunity for each individual in the group to share the experiences they had seen or felt while under the medicines. This is typical of a ceremony: the guide helps interpret the participants' experiences and the messages we received during the ceremony to help us integrate these messages into our daily lives. People shared incredible experiences: visions of family members that had passed without the opportunity to say goodbye, and other deep, meaningful experiences.

I was last. When it was my turn, I answered honestly: I felt gypped. In comparison to the experiences people were sharing, mine was horrible. I told the group how nauseous I'd felt, how out of control, and how isolated and ashamed I felt as a result.

The facilitator asked. "Are you the type of person who typically needs to be in control, and has a problem asking for help?"

"Yes," I answered.

"I wish you would have talked about these experiences while you were having them," the facilitator continued. "We're here for you, to help you and guide you through that."

She was right—I hadn't asked for help. I didn't realize that until she pointed it out.

"You're very hard on yourself," she said.

I told her that I knew that—I just didn't realize it was that apparent. It helped me shift my perspective on my experience.

She went on to explain that my experience hadn't been "horrible;" it was an experience tailored to me and my own body. There was no reason to compare it to another person, because each experience is individualized, and we all perceive our experiences differently. The sick sensations I'd felt were my body's way of purging negative energy and negative stress.

She recommended I watch a movie, *What the Bleep Do We Know!?* to help me understand the visions I'd experienced. The movie dives into quantum physics and discusses different dimensions, and how we typically see in 3D, but that multiple dimensions exist at the same time. The movie also points out that our brain processes 400 billion bits of information a second, but we are only conscious of 2,000 bits. We take in an incredible amount of sensory input, and we cross-check all that data through our own perceptions and filter out patterns that aren't recognizable or familiar. "It's like we're really walking around blind," the facilitator said. When you change those filters of perception, you can begin to see different meanings as a result.

I realized that a huge part of my own personal lens was judgment and bias. I have a history of being very judgmental that connects back to my early attitudes around achievement and how I grew up. The medicines had helped me unleash trauma and repressed stress that had been buried in my subconscious. Slowly, I was seeing how to take on a different lens.

I was beginning to connect the dots and be more connected with people. For a few weeks after my experience, I was on a high, feeling love for nature, and more importantly, for people. I wondered, *am I going to feel like this every day?* This feeling of connection was new for me; I was so used to experiencing other people as my enemies. I went on to have several more experiences, and each one deepened my sense of connection and spirituality.

OPENING THE DOOR TO CONNECTION

One of my more memorable experiences occurred when I felt safe in the environment where the ceremony was held and I had no expectations. In a ceremonial setting, one is often expected to declare an intention prior to ingesting the sacrament. An intention is an aim or goal you want to center your experience around. It can provide an anchor to return to if you find yourself venturing into frightening territory. An intention can be something serious—like to understand the nature of an addiction that's interfering with your life—or it could simply be play, fun, or joy.

My intention before one experience was to forgive and forget any lingering issues that I harbored against my parents. During this specific journey, I remember traveling back in time to my birth. I witnessed myself being born in a hospital to my young parents, my mother nineteen and my father twenty-four. It's difficult to put into words, but I felt the unconditional love my parents had for me as soon as I was placed in their arms after being born.

I could feel how big my parents' hearts were, when accepting me as their own. Witnessing this experience warmed my heart and renewed a sense of love towards my parents. As this dream-like image faded, another image appeared. I was talking to my parents. I saw myself having a conversation with my parents. I heard myself asking, "Why were you so hard on me growing up? Why didn't you love me more and express your love in ways that I needed?" My dad replied, "We did the best we could given the circumstances we were in. We were young adults in a new country with no friends, no family, and no clue how to raise a child. We thought what we were doing was right. All of our actions were out of unconditional love. There was never malicious intent. You were, are, and always will be loved by us."

The next morning, our group gathered around our guide to share our experiences from the night before. When it was my turn to share, I gave a vivid picture, to the best of my memory, of what I saw and heard in my vision. The guide said that now that I have this gift of a message, I should be able to release any disdain or anger against my parents and reframe it. I should be understanding of the predicament they were in and realize that in the end, they are my parents and love me no matter what. Having the guide help reinforce the meaning of my visions really helped me to let go of my anger.

I felt so much lighter in the days and weeks after. I found my personality had shifted. I felt a sense of connection to people that I didn't have before. Was it because my brain chemistry shifted or was it because the rumination had lessened?

My interactions with my parents became more meaningful and I was able to be present with them instead of rehashing old arguments or feeling old unwanted emotions.

One particular day, I went to my parents' house for dinner. I was tired and my dad and I were discussing some needed modifications to their house. I had just gone through a similar modification to my own home and felt what I had to suggest should be taken seriously. Instead, my dad in usual fashion dismissed my perspective and went on to do his own thing.

Normally, I would be triggered, and I would get angry and resentful and the rest of the evening spent at my parents' home would be awkward and in silence. But on this day, I just let the emotion roll off. I was aware of the emotion surfacing, but I held it in check. I was in tune with the turmoil that was going on in my mind, but I consciously decided to stay present in the moment and not let these old emotions of inadequacy surface.

At that moment, I remembered my message from my magic mushroom experience: that my parents love me regardless of who I am or what I've done. Instead of arguing or having a scowl on my face, I simply accepted the circumstances for what they were and didn't analyze it any further. I didn't ruminate over this like I normally do, nor did I dwell on this for days after. I stayed present.

On another day leaving my parents home, they extended a hug. Growing up, these hugs or other overt signs of affection were not the norm. My parents now will hug us, but it's a weird side-hug. They don't hug in the frontal plane. Whenever they initiated a side hug, I'd always think in the back of my head that this was fake and ingenuine because it wasn't what I wanted or how I thought a hug should be expressed.

On this day, I told myself, "It's a hug. Accept it for what it is and enjoy it. It's their way of expressing their unconditional love for me. It's unique and it's from my parents. How could I second guess this intention?" This revelation was spawned by my psychedelic experience, which I was integrating into my daily life. I'll always be indebted to the wisdom the plant medicine provided me that night.

Over the ensuing month, I noticed that I also was more open-minded, curious, and even more imaginative. My experience is not uncommon: a study in 2011 demonstrated that those who participated in experiences occasioned by psilocybin often showed increases in aesthetic appreciation, imagination, and creativity. In fact, one year after the study, the personality trait of openness still remained above baseline in individuals participating in the study.[59]

USING PSYCHEDELICS TO FORGE CONNECTIONS

Anyone who is looking for meaning in their life can benefit from exploration with psychedelics because their purpose is to give you a sensation of connection with the universe and with other people. Research has shown a connection between the use of psychedelics and improved emotional

---

59   Katherine A. MacLean, Matthew W. Johnson, and Roland R. Griffiths, "Mystical Experiences Occasioned by the Hallucinogen Psilocybin Lead to Increases in the Personality Domain of Openness," *Journal of Psychopharmacology*, September 28, 2011.

stability, fewer symptoms of anxiety and depression, and greater levels of spirituality.[60]

In my case, the traumas in my life had made me more introverted and isolated, and psychedelics have helped me open myself up a little more each time. My goal is to continue to do psychedelics until I feel I have put aside my distrust toward people and have a feeling of connectivity driving my desire to meet people. That's what the universe is all about and what we as humans are meant to do, whether we're connecting through our experiences of trauma or joy. Psychedelics are an efficient way of accomplishing my goals without having to endure endless hours of psychotherapy. These medicines do so much in so little time.

INTEGRATING YOUR EXPERIENCE

If you choose to do psychedelic-assisted therapy, it's important to do it under a guide or facilitator to help integrate the day after the experience, as well as continuously in the weeks and months that follow. It's hard to gain a full perspective of your experience on your own; you will usually need a trained professional to help you process the feelings and emotions that come up.

---

60 American Psychological Association, "Can Psychedelic Drugs Heal?" *Science Daily,* August 9, 2018.

Your guide will help shape the way you think during the journey and help you through the experiences you may have.

Over the experiences I've had so far, I've had multiple facilitators, and my experience with each was very different. I felt safe with the first facilitator and was confident that I would be guided through whatever visions I had. The other facilitators had good intentions, but their lack of experience or specific methods and different personalities didn't gel with me. If you're going to go through a psychedelic experience to process trauma and better yourself as a human being, there are several important factors to consider:

1. You need to make sure you're in a safe, comfortable environment.
2. If you're with others, make sure they're people you're comfortable with as you go through these intimate experiences.
3. You should have an experienced facilitator that you trust. Seek out referrals from people you trust.
4. It's important to have a positive mindset. The mood you have going into the session can influence your experience.

Psychedelics aren't a "quick fix," but they do change your brain chemistry in a positive way. They enhance neuroplasticity, allowing us to create new connections in our brains as well as repair old and damaged ones. This explains why positive changes in mood and brain function persist even after the acute effects of the drug have subsided.[61]

I began my exploration into psychedelics with a goal: I wanted to discover my purpose. These experiences have helped to point me in a direction and light my path. They can help you tap into your inner guidance. It can be beneficial to follow up with a psychotherapist experienced in psychedelics who can help you process your experiences and continue with your spiritual enlightenment.

PRACTICING SELFLESSNESS AND TRUE CONNECTION

Ultimately, my experiences have helped me be more present, more connected to myself, and more connected to other people. I learned that I am doing the universe a disservice when I am not fully present with people. My judgment of others and of myself had caused me to retract and retreat into my own isolation. My distrust had caused me to lose my sense of presence with other people.

You can tell when someone is listening and truly present; you can see it in their eyes. I now try hard to do that for people. There are many gifts we can give to others—financial giving

---

61 Ly Calvin, et al, "Psychedelics Promote Structural and Functional Neural Plasticity," *Cell Reports*, June 12, 2018, 23(22): 3170-3182.

is a common example—but the biggest gift you can give to someone is being present with them.

Psychedelics have helped me shed my judgment, and in that process, I've become more mindful, with non-judgmental moment-to-moment awareness.

Now, four years into my remission, I've begun to understand how to shape my path for the present and for the future.

CONCLUSION

At the time of this writing, I had my five-year anniversary of my diagnosis. The quality of my life has changed dramatically in that time, and some of the biggest impacts have been the most subtle.

A group of my college friends gets together once a year to hang out and watch our alma mater play basketball. A few years ago, this experience would have filled me with anxiety. I would ruminate in judgmental thoughts: *They're still stuck in the same rambunctious behavior. I can't wait for this night to be over. Why am I here?* I would have conversations with people, and I could see they felt disconnected from me. I would drink myself into oblivion to keep up with these guys, wishing the whole time that I could just escape.

This year was different. I had my fair share of drinks (moderation includes falling off the wagon every once in a while), but I didn't feel like I needed to escape. I *wanted* to be present. I was enjoying having conversations with my friends. I felt a sense of connectedness that I didn't have before.

I can't remember the last time I felt that way—maybe it was in college, or even earlier, as a little kid, before secondary thoughts and judgments would come into my head, when I took everything people said for what it was, and I experienced people for who they were and that's all there was.

The judgments I had—for myself and for others—created physical stress on my body. Constant rumination is exhausting and alienating. When we can connect to a feeling of belonging, we reduce stress and create positive effects not only for our minds but in our physical health.

In these moments, with my friends, I glimpsed how life can be when I live moment to moment.

I'm experiencing a new normal in the health of my mind, body, and spirit. So often, the lifestyles we build alienate us from our own needs and from the people around us. We experience disconnection from our bodies, our relationships, and our spirituality. But these three crucial areas of our lives can improve when we connect back to our own self-care.

Explore your curiosity. Whether you're interested in improving your physical well-being, your mental well-being, or your spiritual well-being, look for ways you can develop your awareness. Whether it's as simple as becoming more conscious of the foods you put into your body, or as complex as taking a spiritual journey with psychedelics, take your next step with an open mind, and pay attention to the large and subtle shifts that result.

When you find a new practice that enhances your life—one that you learn from this book, or one you discover in your own experience—make it a routine. This is how we change the world, little by little. The small improvements we make get multiplied when we turn them into daily habits and share them with others.

As a healthcare provider, I took an oath to help humanity. There is so much illness in this world that can be prevented or treated with the tenets in this book. As you find practices that work for you, that help you heal and feel fully present and alive, find one person to pay it forward to.

When we are of service to others, we fuel our collective connection to the universe, and to our own health and vibrancy within it.

ABOUT THE
AUTHOR

DR. DIVA NAGULA has been a physician for over twenty years. His proactive mentality during his battle with cancer led him to pursue further training in integrative medicine at the University of Arizona under the renowned Andrew Weil, MD. Integrative medicine, a blend of traditional and alternative medicine, gave Dr. Nagula the tools to help heal his mind, body, and spirit during his cancer battle. Those tools also help him maintain his health now that he's in remission. Dr. Nagula recently moved to the greater Washington, DC area where he is close to his family and friends and owns and operates an on-demand intravenous hydration concierge business.

Made in the USA
Middletown, DE
03 December 2019

79913438R00120